LOVE'S PURSUIT

Journey to Wellness

D. B. MARSHALL, MSW

For information, contact Love's Pursuit Publishing or info@lovespursuitatl.net

The information and opinions expressed in this book are for educational and informational purposes only and are not intended as medical, psychiatric, or psychological advice, diagnosis, or treatment. Please consult with a personal physician or other health care professional for your specific mental and/or physical health care needs or concerns. No physician-patient relationship is created by reading this book. Do not avoid or delay seeking medical advice or attention from your health care provider because of something you read or learned about in this book. If you are experiencing an emergency, seek appropriate medical attention immediately. If you are suffering from depression, hopelessness, or thoughts of suicide, please call the **National Suicide Prevention Lifeline** *at 1-800-273-TALK or 1-800-273-8255,* mentalhealth.gov, drugabuse.gov, *and* samosa.gov.

Cover design by OLaLa Merkel

Printed and bound in the United States of America

The Library of Congress has established a record for this title.

Love's Pursuit: Journey to Wellness / D.B. Marshall. — 1st ed.
ISBN 978-1-7359852-0-6

DEDICATION

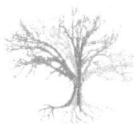

To my grandfather, grandmother, father, mother, uncles, aunts, and siblings, who are the greatest gifts Heaven has showered me with and given so much love and care. Your support has brought me through uncomfortable, depressive valleys and elevated me onto countless mountain tops. For this, I THANK YOU!

To my A-list celebrities, though we have never met, you have saved my life. As I write this dedication, the memories of you during my traumatic experience flood my eyes, causing a rush of emotion and tears. Each teardrop represents 3% water and 97% positive emotions. I have sung and danced with you; my heart laughed and cried with you, and because without you, I am not sure where I would be. You lifted me; therefore, I HONOR YOU! YOU SAVED MY LIFE!

Tisha Campbell | *Little Shop of Horrors, Rags to Riches, School Daze, Push, and Martin*

Tichina Arnold | *Little Shop of Horrors and Martin*

Michelle Weeks | *Little Shop of Horrors*

Dolly Parton | *Best Little Whorehouse in Texas, 9 to 5, and Joyful Noise*

Patti Labelle | *The Bluebells, Labelle, and Patti Labelle albums, A Different World, and Out All Night*

Earvin "*Magic*" Johnson | *Talent, skills, and legacy. The first African American male I heard about owning a business that gave back to the community. He opened a movie theatre in Greenbrier Mall in Atlanta, GA*

Taraji P. Henson | *Mental Health Campaign and Awareness*

Destiny's Child | *The Writing's on the Wall through Destiny Fulfilled. My Journey to Wellness and self-discovery traveled with you. After fulfilling a challenge, I ask God what's next.*

RuPaul & Drag Race Family | *I am a RU fan. I find solace in your art, creativity, and positive messages. I binge-watch every season all year round. It always feels like Christmas watching you.*

Ellen Degeneres | *Because of you, I laugh and smile when I think I no longer have a reason to laugh or smile. Because of you, I no longer require a sprinkler system to water my grass; I just use my tears.*

ACKNOWLEDGMENTS

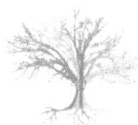

This book would not have manifested without the outpouring support, assistance, and encouragement of so many beautiful souls. I am indebted to the incredible **Love's Pursuit** faithful followers who believed in me when I did not.

Chief among my support team is Mr. Harper, who dealt with the twists and turns, and there were more of those than I would have liked to have experienced. Sometimes space and silence are precisely what is needed to reset, and I was given those options.

I am also grateful for each soul mentioned in the book. Their stories help breathe life into the project. They understood what it meant to me. They opened their hearts and homes to help bring awareness, normalize these issues, and support communities worldwide. There were times I became disheartened because of the stress, barriers, and disappointments, but they showed up every time with happy feet and luminous smiles that lit up the room to support one of my dreams.

Special Thank You
Dr. D. Pulley | J. Fleming | G. Daigle | D. Safford
J. Brogdon | L. Zephir | Mrs. Williams | M. Rouse
D. Dykes (my Shonny) | Mrs. Van Beverhart

FOREWORD

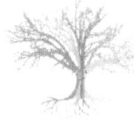

I have been a Spiritual Leader for over 30 years and a mental health professional for 23 years. I have worked with hundreds of people worldwide in individual, couple, family, and group counseling and therapeutic workshops. I often look for books that parishioners and clients alike can read outside of the sessions to reinforce the work that we do in the sessions. This book is one that I will add to my resource guide for individuals to utilize. It is about real people with real issues, and it provides real solutions that anyone can use.

D.B. Marshall is utterly vulnerable in his vignettes. He allows the reader into his sacred space. They walk with him hand-in-hand along his wholeness path and **Love's Pursuit**. He shares his process of unfoldment and invites us to grow in our healing process as well.

Not only does D.B. Marshall share his *Journey to Wellness* story, but he also gives other people who have been through similar experiences the opportunity to provide their perspectives. The common ground in all the anecdotes is that they use the cognitive-behavioral process of recovery, which addresses the unity of our thoughts, feelings, and actions. They also integrate positive psychology and wellness practices such as journaling and affirmations for holistic growth and development.

Regardless of age, race, gender, orientation, socioeconomic status, criminal background, family dynamic, educational level, religion, and culture, anyone who reads these stories and utilizes these tools can learn to live a holistically healthy, balanced, and well-rounded life. The truth principles espoused in this book are universal and will work if you work them. They will increase your self-image, self-esteem, and self-worth and help you to discover your destiny. As we become better as individuals, we can lift the universe's vibration and the earth's energy to create a planet that works for everyone.

– Dr. Doral R. Pulley, LCPC-S
Author, *Prayer: Your Spiritual Toolbox*

Contents

PART FIVE

PART SIX

PART SEVEN

PART EIGHT

PART NINE

INTRODUCTION

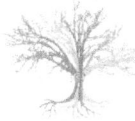

Take a moment and think about how much time you have invested in grade school, undergraduate and graduate programs, art and music careers, and other areas of your life you have mastered. Which of these has afforded you true and lasting happiness and fulfillment? Now, query yourself about how much time you have invested in your healing and your wholeness and answer honestly. Are you perhaps worse off despite all these conventional trainings? Tell me, how many hours in a week have you participated in uninterrupted self-love ventures? In doing so, awareness increases, which also boosts laughter, self-love, empowerment, and tranquility.

Humans are tripartite beings, meaning we are composed of three parts: spirit, soul, and body, with the mind as the coordinating faculty. We experience misery and joylessness when any one of these is in turmoil. Wholeness in being is achieved when all components are in harmony. Adversity happens on all levels except one—the spirit. The spirit is whole. It is also healthy. Not only that, but it can also be said to be the powerhouse. Therefore, we seek and draw from the strength of spirit to assist us through our journey to live a happy, fulfilled life.

Everyone desires happiness, for *a merry heart doeth good like a medicine.* Happiness stems from a sense of fulfillment. The greatest fulfillment is the fulfillment of our life's purpose. This begins with the awareness and understanding that each one of us is born with a great purpose. In other words, everyone's existence has its ultimate significance. It is not by chance that we woke up this morning healthy. It is to fulfill a purpose and thereby tell our stories. Our stories go a long way to inspire and revitalize our world. We have been given a voice to communicate precisely what we feel, why we feel, and how we feel. And every word we speak, whether formal or informal, is potent with a quantum of energy and power.

Words have the power to invigorate Humanity with Humility, Hope, Happiness, and Honor. Given the power words possess, we must pause, process, and respond accurately when we speak, with the intention and hope to heal our brothers and sisters and not deliberately hurt them. Though we cannot control what people say, we can manage how we respond to what is said. However, we can influence others by modeling positive thoughts and behaviors. Who gives words power? We do! That is right, my friend. Without us, words are simply words. We give power to what we say by our choice of words, tone of voice, wishes in our minds, and more. Each word begins with a thought. From that thought (in the mind), we decide if that word would result in an action or inaction (in the body). Oh, but wait, it does not stop there! The action or inaction proceeds to drive our soul journey. As we can see, the mind, body, and soul constantly communicate with one another. It is a continuous journey that can either be a vicious or virtuous cycle. You choose.

As you read **Love's Pursuit**: *Journey to Wellness*, you will explore different ways to make a deeper connection with the "self" and successfully jumpstart your self-discovery odyssey—Your Purpose. Research tells us it takes approximately two months—**66 days, to be exact**—to change or adopt a new behavior. Not only is the behavior adopted, but it becomes automatic. It becomes our muscle memory and responds on its own as an involuntary action. This is akin to other autonomous functions of our body, like the beating of the heart or even breathing. We encourage readers to commit and invest a minimum of **66 days**—although we recommend **99 days**–to this journey of self-discovery. Do this by asking the tough questions, which include *what, when, where,* but more importantly, *why* and *how.* In doing so, you will affirm, cultivate, and align the soul properly and transform your life. When you connect and align with your soul daily, life no longer feels like a fight or a struggle. To develop strong connections, one must adopt and practice positive communication. I refer to this as restructuring thoughts through a creative art expression that consists of a steady and smooth communication flow. The communication flow is simply thought patterns that determine how you interact with yourself and others. For instance, if you work in a hostile work environment, it is very likely the environment will eventually cause feelings of fear, nervousness, anxiety, and defensive reactions or responses. You will find yourself spiraling out of control like the domino effect. This results in one thing falling, causing the downfall of multiple other things. Like a virus, the negativity will transmit. Like cancer, it will metastasize and infect family, friends, and innocent bystanders, even the cashier at the checkout line!

It is imperative to take time out for yourself—just you—and invest in your healing and transformation process. It is possible! The *Journey to Wellness* stories of individuals highlighted in the book are testimonies that support this notion. You can start by reading them. Like you, they have lived through chaos, found their voices, persevered, and are prevailing. Throughout the book, there are activities to encourage supportive reflections to help identify and cope with underlying cognitive and emotional distress. The objective is to comfort, advise, encourage, and reassure "self" and pave the way for other travelers. It is actively listening with **Intention** and giving **Attention** to the person, place, or thing deserving of your time and **Attention.**

The book infuses cognitive-behavioral and positive psychology theories and utilizes each model to breakdown **Love's Pursuit:** *Journey to Wellness* stories. The cognitive-

3

behavioral model is based on the concept of our thoughts (cognitive), our feelings (emotion), and our actions or inaction (behavior) rolled into one. Again, our thoughts determine our emotional and behavioral reactions and responses. Positive psychology complements cognitive-behavioral theory by focusing on character strengths and behaviors, which encourage individuals to develop a purposeful life—to move beyond merely existing to living and having a meaningful, fulfilling experience. Self-help activities are also presented throughout the book to help change negative thoughts into positive ones. Some of the techniques are self-talks, affirmations, guided discovery, questions, journaling, and situational exposures.

The book also shares the participants' stories using the models and D.B. Marshall's personal experiences to break down and simplify each experience. The objective is to present and facilitate the information in a way the readers can identify signs and symptoms of negative thoughts, trauma, and other cognitive challenges. Please note the participants volunteered their time and attention and only provided information that they were comfortable sharing. These individuals have done the work, and now it is your time. Are you ready? Let us establish new standards and re-establish a new personal order inclusive of revised tasks, values, beliefs, and morals. **You are worth it!**

We are so delighted you chose us to take this journey with, and we look forward to seeing and hearing how the book inspired your *Journey to Wellness*. Please share your stories on our social media platforms [*@lovespursuitatl*], as you may be featured in our next wellness project. Your journey starts here, starts now, so let us begin!

Take a deep breath and hold it for three seconds, then exhale. Repeat it two more times. After completing all three inhales and exhales, recite the following affirmations and repeat three more times. One for the mind, for the body, and the soul.

- **I usher out the old**; therefore, I release the hurt, pain, disappointments, and erroneous ideas and beliefs.

- **I make room for the new**—new love, refreshing love, self-love, and lasting love.
- **I connect with the spirit** as it is whole, and it is necessary to deepen and balance my mind, soul, and body for future endeavors.

It is official! Your **Love's Pursuit**: *Journey to Wellness* has begun. Keep in mind, you must make it happen by being consistent if you desire change, happiness, and transformation.

Oh, and by the way, if no one has told you that they love you today, please allow me to be the first: I love you!

D.B. Marshall
Atlanta, Georgia

PART ONE

Understanding Negativity and Negative Thoughts

A negative, hostile, and obsessive internal dialogue generates the feeling of being in a black hole. The light goes out and the hopes, one by one, disappear. Learning to turn negative thoughts into positive ones is more than just a want; it is a need that produces healthy coping mechanisms to survive and thrive. Once the decision is made to fight another day, practical tools must be accessible to continue to live despite the danger, trauma, or hardship. The tools are designed to assist the "set-up" to the "step-forth" into the breakthrough. It means the planning and developing phases are activated to prosper, be fortunate and successful, grow, and vigorously flourish into the most beautiful parts of you.

We all have negative thoughts that bounce around in our minds. At a certain point, they may raise their voices and send us clear messages: "you are nobody, you will never make it, you will fail, no matter how hard you try, it will always end the same." We are human, and our minds tend to drift much more often than we would like. This unedifying rumination process has been referred to by neuroscientists as "bias of negativity."

1

Emotional psychology experts argue it is permissible to have up to three negative thoughts a day. It is not a question of closing our eyes to reality or building walls in the face of difficulties, fears, and worries. The key lies in not letting ourselves be stopped by these thought patterns in which, almost without realizing it, we prevent the entry of resilience, triumph, motivation, or personal growth.

As discovered by the famous neuroimaging laboratory of the University of California, each of us has up to 70,000 thoughts a day. And yes, a large portion of them are negative, limiting, and frustrating. But in the face of this intrusive and, at times, compelling presence, we have the option at our disposal to accept and transform them.

Changing certain mental patterns is difficult but not impossible if you put the necessary effort into it. It is not enough to eliminate negative thoughts every now and then; you have to try to replace them with positive ideas whenever the opportunity arises. The human brain does indeed have a predilection for negativity but is elastic enough to change its habits, as long as you dare to insist. It is essential to maintain a positive attitude towards any situation because it is a way to keep moving forward no matter how difficult it seems. First, it is vital to understand negative thoughts are crucial in determining future outcomes. So why is the struggle so real?

Struggles with Negative Thoughts

The struggle is real! As previously stated, researchers argue that we experience up to 70,000 thoughts a day, of which most are negative. Therefore, it is important for us to learn how to manage negative thoughts as they are the main cause of suffering. For example, if I think about a bad moment in my life, a negative emotion is produced, which causes feelings of pain or distress. If, on the other hand, I think of a pleasant experience in my life, I

2

feel a positive emotion which produces joy. Remembering a thousand times when our partners left us or what we could have said to our bosses when they fired us, for example, does not help us overcome adverse situations. It only repurposes feelings that are not so positive, creating a problematic vicious cycle to break. It is like our minds are at civil war, occupied continuously and distracted by these thoughts, fighting internal battles, leaving little to no room to plant positive seeds for new growth.

Do you know and can you identify your Nemesis? Your Nemesis's thoughts are those that separate us from ourselves and others: antipathy, distrust, suspicion, resentment, hatred, jealousy, envy, cruelty, anger, anxiety, agitation, greed, and more. In comparison, the Superhero or heroic thoughts create a union with others and are sympathy, trust, kindness, forgiveness, love, understanding, compassion, generosity solidarity, calm, patience, flexibility, gratitude, and the like. In short, negative thoughts represent the loss of trust and love and cause fear of living, while positive thoughts are the reflection of trust and love and, therefore, the absence of fear. Fear is precisely the absence of love to trust in one's own strength. However, we must immediately point out that only the excess of fear is pathological because it is normal, useful, and essential to feeling fear, perhaps even a strong suspicion, in the face of real dangers.

Scientists have found that we tend to have a penchant for the negative. There is a good and healthy reason for this; our brains usually react more strongly to a negative stimulus than to a positive impulse of the same strength. Such a response is necessary to ensure our survival. Unfortunately, excessive fear almost always derives from imaginary dangers or from exaggerating threats that occur in the presence of a fragile ego.

The fundamental difference between negative and positive thoughts is the former is involuntary or spontaneous (i.e., automatic), while positive thoughts are voluntary and

3

therefore require an effort on our part to produce and reproduce them until they are embedded in our minds and overshadow the negative and regenerate automatically. Furthermore, negative thoughts are often compulsive or constricting and therefore are neurotic in nature, caused by maladjustment to the environment. It must also be said that negative thoughts, coming directly from the unconscious or instinctive self, are in stark contrast to our conscious and rational parts (otherwise, they would not be negative).

These recurring thoughts indicate something happened in our lives, and we become fearful of the unknown. If the "happened" repeats itself and happens again, could we survive it a second time? Or would we capitulate to the negative forces arrayed against us and signed the Nemesis's list of demands? For me, fear is a disease. It propagates if it is not contained. The fear of getting sick, the obsession with having everything under control at home and at work, or the fear of the declining health of loved ones are thoughts down the yellow brick road to tragedy. There are many unproductive thoughts that can constantly crowd our minds.

In the long run, this vicious cycle can lead to much more severe consequences, such as depression, panic attacks, substance addiction, or eating disorders. In fact, obsessive thoughts do not make room for positive growth; you do! These embedded images in our intricate world of feelings, sensations, and behaviors lead to obsessive thinking. Our minds begin to lose traction, grip, and control over recurring, distressing thoughts and images perpetuating pessimism at its peak. Moreover, this cycle moves us away from having a solution-focused approach: the mind focuses on the problems and not on its solution.

However, it is important to know even negative thoughts, as well as the emotions that arise from them, can prove useful in any given circumstance. Even anger can be useful in some instances. And obliterating it would be a very bad business because we would no longer know how to defend ourselves from others' ill-intention and abuse. Ultimately, any human trait is only harmful when it becomes excessive. As always, it is too much that cripples.

Causes of Negative Thoughts

Having intrusive thoughts is more common than you think. As human beings, our minds fabricate thousands of thoughts over the days that come to us in very different ways. They can be reflections and ideas that bring us fruit, as well as thoughts that are distinct and foreign to what we consider to be expected.

The manifestations of these thoughts are endless and can take on thematic representations that may or may not make immediate sense to the people who have them. Some deal with negative images of reality, others with terrifying ideas; an unlimited variety of themes is possible. Sometimes, intrusive thoughts like these arise in us precisely because we do not want to act or think this way, as they are simply the most inappropriate thing our mind can imagine. Having that kind of thinking is possible and normal at some point in our lives.

Positive intrusive thoughts are spontaneous ideas and reflections we have throughout life that can also persist in our minds. In these cases, the themes can also be diverse, but they arouse nothing but pleasures and healthy questions by not attacking us. Everyday situations, conversations with friends, a life partner, different environments, a trip—these and other examples of events can awaken beneficial insights in our minds. The objective is to connect with them until we understand and reap their rewards. Negative intrusive thoughts are closely linked to fear. Despite being an absolutely natural and healthy feeling whose function is to protect us from major problems and difficulties, it ends up becoming something irrational and destructive, limiting our ability to think, act, and feel free of our desires.

The fears caused by these thoughts can represent a great deal of angst. Still, they gain a much greater dimension when the person mistakenly evaluates them as having a greater probability of happening, continuing to develop the obsessions and difficulties that normally accompany them. We tend to be unaware of them because we are not aware of ourselves. Other times, they bother us, as they are not aligned with our morals, values, and beliefs. The more we avoid such thoughts or worry about them, the more present and insistent they become in our minds. Not wanting to think about something already makes us think about it. By giving such importance to these thoughts, we greatly increase the risk of repeatedly having them. This book will further explain that negative thought, or any thought for that matter, influences who we are, what we represent, and who we are becoming.

Effects of Negative Thoughts

Thoughts become intruders and, if we think about them too much, they end up becoming obsessions that limit our actions. The need to mull over what worries us can arise in any situation while we are working, shopping, or brushing our teeth. Without realizing it, they can occupy our minds, also affecting our mood.

These thoughts feed and support the relentless cycle and create negative consequences in people's lives. For example, if Teresa is obsessing over producing a perfect work product, she will likely never be satisfied and neglect other areas of her life, causing an imbalance. This is not healthy. Listen, I know exactly what never satisfied feels and looks like because I entertained a relationship with someone who was never satisfied. An unsatisfied individual is always in pursuit of provisional happiness to avoid dealing with the real issue. This pseudo happiness is

6

temporary until the next victim knocks on their door. They will always "think" people and objects will fill a void, when in fact, they must find happiness on their own and deep within. It starts with demystifying negative thoughts and reprogramming the mind. If you are uncertain of the consequences of negative thoughts, here are a few to consider:

- **Phobic avoidance**—This is a situation that causes fear. We may avoid leaving the house, driving the car, touching objects we consider dirty, etc. This limits our daily lives and prevents us from living and enjoying the beauties of the world.

- **Repeatedly checking**—This is a typical compulsion of obsession. When we close the door of the house or car and verify ten times that it is closed, we are putting into practice a compulsion that calms us at the moment but which, in reality, perpetuates anxiety and obsessions.

- **Procrastination**—The thought "I will do it another day" can end up making it impossible for us to carry out our activities.

- **Need for perfection**—Perfection is the enemy of good, and for this reason, you could lose the sense of things to obtain something impossible—for example, Teresa's obsession with perfecting her work.

- **Heart attack risk**—According to researchers from the Department of Psychiatry at Päijät-Häme Central Hospital, Finland, through 11 years of research involving 2,267 people aged between 52 and 76, pessimism could lead to severe heart diseases such as inflammation and heart attacks.

- **Depression**—Thinking negatively may lead the person to give up more easily when experiencing difficulties or adversity. Constant ruminating can shape our worldview and produce a pessimistic perception.

- **Anxiety and panic attacks**—The fear of dying or failing to attribute to pessimism can become chronic and increase anxiety levels to the point of leading to panic attacks. The risk is falling prey to a pool of insecurities from which, over time, it is increasingly difficult to emerge.
- **Compromises personal relationships**—Whether they are friends, partners, or relatives, thinking negatively and finding something wrong with every action, even towards others, could isolate us and foment anger towards us and frustration within us.
- **Compromises working relationships**—Even on the working level, the risk is to look like the classic bird of ill omen. Telling your boss you are unwilling or unable to achieve a goal is always an action to avoid. The risk is losing your job and being unpleasant and unwilling to take the initiative, especially if you work as a team.
- **Increases the sense of loneliness**—Constantly complaining and seeing everything as hopeless can isolate "self" from others at the behest of others. Nobody likes to have a person by their side who only remembers risks and vicissitudes. One can give the idea of being inconclusive people and little inclined to change.

Moving Away from the World of Negativity to Positivity
When destructive thoughts flood the mind, it is good to change your attitude and learn to relativize and avoid falling into the vortex of negativity. Changing negative thinking or thoughts is not easy, but it becomes easier to remember that positive thinking or thoughts are based on creating positive experiences. Our thoughts are based on experiences, feelings, and emotions we

have lived in the past. You can change your thinking by having a similar positive experience, with the intent it will strike differently from the last time. Experience is the key to changing our thoughts and perspectives. So if you want to change your thoughts and reality consciously, be the creator you were born to be, and create experiences that will rewrite or reprogram those not-so-good moments. It does not matter that they have not happened yet: explore, execute, and make them real. Take action. Actors are charged with playing many character roles, thus creating experiences to appease the viewer. Remember, you have the lead role; therefore, control the narrative by changing your circumstance from problem-centered to solution-focused. This is your screenplay titled **Love's Pursuit:** *Journey to Wellness*, Take One!

Journey

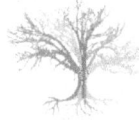

Proclaim:

*My journey to wellness is not a sprint but a process.
Therefore, I will manage my inner conflicts and
trust myself more to enjoy life's journey.*

One thing for sure is that storms come, and storms go. Though it does not usually seem like they will pass, eventually, they do. There are moments when two or more storms form concurrently in the atmosphere, and another is approaching landfall—all at once. What is even more appalling, sometimes they strategically hit in the same area as if it were marked for destruction.

Have you felt like you could not catch a breather? You find your situation rapidly changing—for the worse and worst—thus forcing you to run into the hayloft for safety because there is no bunker in sight, and you cannot afford to build one at the moment. The storm happens so fast that taking-a-deep-breath becomes useless. Calling for succor or trying to assess the situation are unavailable options. I have yet to meet anyone who celebrates or appreciates their storms. The reason is that storms create turmoil and have the potential of causing severe damage. I believe it is a risk most would not like to endure.

Storms are made up of many facets. They manifest physically, mentally, and emotionally. Based on the fierceness of the storm and your condition, it can leave a lasting and unforgettable impact, ranging from homelessness to feelings of helplessness, despondency, depression, suicide, and other ills in between. My own storms resulted from overwhelming stress, which exceeded my ability to cope, resulting in frustration, anxiety, and depression. Though such experiences can be traumatic, my journey to wellness showed me that it is not the storm that puts us in a state of confusion. It was my reaction to the storm—inner conflict—that created the turmoil. What are your storms? How did you react during the stormy weather? Did you run, hide, or take cover? Did you attack, or did you weather the storm? Hopefully, our stories will assist you in approaching storms more positively.

In the beginning, my responses were diplomatic, and they were always considerate of people. However, when I felt used, manipulated, and unfulfilled, my positive approach shifted to a defensive one. My behaviors became less responsive and more reactive. Was that the best choice? No, it was not. You will know the difference and the best choice to make when you understand that the storms are not really about the people involved. The truth is that I could have responded instead of reacting. From this experience, I conclude there is a difference between "reaction" and "response." A reaction is usually an action performed without thinking or processing. It is an immediate, unconscious return of actions charged with beliefs, biases, and prejudices seeking to survive an attack. The goal is to protect oneself irrespective of the health of others. On the other hand, responsiveness is driven by logical thought processes; it is a joint effort of one's consciousness and unconsciousness to consider oneself and all those involved.

The goal is to cause minimal damage while staying true to oneself. Knowing the difference will assist with your wellness journey. Again, it is a process. It is a holistic, continuous approach towards change, in the manner calculated most appropriate. Which approach do you prefer, the reaction or the response? Remember, reactions create more and more hostilities.

I have stated my reactions—inner conflict—created turmoil; it led to despair when it was beyond the bounds of my capacity. Mismanaging the storms blocked dreams, started nightmares, and caused unhappy feelings. I found myself more introspective, not necessarily responding to others but more focused on responding to myself. Initially, I accepted there was no return on my investment—the time and energy spent. The only person who has access to manage and calm the storm is me. To gain clarity, conscious and unconscious thoughts were scheduled to negotiate. Intuition and logic were to sit across the table to dialogue. When I recognized this was nonexistent, I requested annual leave from work and began dealing with the inner conflict. When I committed myself to do the work, the confusion was supplanted by potential. Precious memories began to spring in my mind, which evoked smiles and delight in my life. What issued from that is more than enough energy to carry me through and weather the storms. Two things are at work here: hope and potential.

Hope can be harvested from precious memories— maybe about a childhood dream, a promise, an initial resolve, a morale-inducing story, and so forth. Potential motivates you to realize you have what it takes to respond and not react to the storm and prevail.

It is my desire that you recognize your potential— everyone has at least one or two. Armed with the awareness of your potentials, confidently assert, "I am excellence personified. This is not the best version of me, for my skill set is still developing, and my best self is still evolving."

Hope and Potential are two valuable tools worth adding to your journey kit. They will prove invaluable during the storms. Potential stirs up the genius within, while hope enables you to endure suffering without complaining as you strive for greatness. *"Potential looks for greatness while hope is patiently working to develop the greatness you found."*

To be true, suffering in hope is no easy task nor is patiently waiting for the incubation of the life to which you look forward. Life storms are often unforeseen and can have you traveling down an unpredictable arduous path. At this point, it begins to appear as if you are abandoned and have lost your achievements. When the gravity of storms is immense and its frequency high, one seems to find no safe haven in which to anchor. You feel hopeless and abandoned due to a developing negative perception of yourself, especially when you recall so-called golden opportunities that slipped through your fingertips. How many opportunities do you feel you have flushed down the toilet? But let me let you in on a secret: when you begin to experience feelings of this sort and magnitude, it is an indication you are worthy and capable of a better life, a change from the status quo. It is for you to long for more, to seek for more. What is the "more" you seek? The "more" here symbolizes potential expansion. Your soul is pursuing deeper love, higher levels of consciousness, and spiritual awakening.

In order to know the "more" you seek, first, you must identify the inner conflict that requires managing. Is it related to sex, morals, ego, values, self-image, or love, or is it "meta" in nature? There are more types of conflicts, and these inner conflicts must be identified and dealt with because they constitute clogs in the wheel of your journey. They hinder your progression in seeking for the "more." This activity will help complete the inner work and assist you in trusting your decisions. This may also require you to take a break or terminate a non-rewarding relationship, project, or career path that made you smile in the past but only now restricts your potential. (With most things we are passionate about, we become emotionally vested in them and give 150%.) It will challenge you in ways unimaginable. It will make the difference in your life in times of storms, whether you will give in to the disheartening situation or remain steadfast.

But . . . you know, I like to say "but" with emphasis and a short pause whenever I am speaking. And when I write, I like to put a comma beside it; like (,) but after the storms is a soiree; (,) but after the pain is a party. There is great intention behind that, however. This is because it is an independent clause in preparation for a breakthrough. It makes the difference between hope and anxiety, optimism and pessimism, success and failure, victory and defeat, and response and reaction.

Hope says, I did not expect the sickness, but I am recuperating. Anxiety says, I am recuperating, but I am still sick. "Comma or (,) but" means a change is happening or is about to happen. Something new is in the offing. Learn to use your buts and use them well. For me, the word sends chills traveling down from my head to my feet—a sign of the good change I anticipate in my journey through the midst of the storms. I hope you feel the same.

Make no mistake about this; everyone faces storms at one point or another in their life. If you do not have any now, wait and keep living, for one is sure to come soon. It is not a curse but a fact about life. Despite our efforts, things can turn out differently. We feel as if our blood, sweat, and tears have been lived in vain. We are left emotionally disoriented and spiraling out of control because the outcome is different than expected. What happens next? Where do you go? How do you face the unsavory change? The embarrassment alone inflames reactions and aggressive behaviors that once lay dormant. What are your choices? Ask yourself, "Do I choose reaction for instant gratification, or choose response and suffer through the pain?" Choose you! Choose more! Choose wellness!

I have not been the best at terminating emotional investments, but I have improved over the years. I used to describe myself as long-suffering: the man who has endured prolonged challenges because I saw (and still see) the good in people instead of only the good in me; the man who supported them through adversity without yielding, patiently waiting for my turn to shine; the man who stood behind the scenes cheering the greedy, honing their talents and seeing them progress year after year until they no longer chose me.

When you are successful at duplicating your recipe in others, this is when life becomes clear to you. The clarity unveils that you are confident you are on the right track of the journey to purpose. This is when you send a personal invitation to yourself—a self-RSVP—for the soiree. The invitation reads, "You are cordially invited to Restoration, Happiness, Contentment, and Fulfillment."

At the party, there are two entities rejoining: the body and soul. They boogie with joy and contentment, celebrating even the reckoning of the "unfulfillment" and long-suffering. Though material gains and abundance may seem depleted, accomplishment and experience brought us through the storms. It is a celebration of completion, a sense of wholeness. Stress is released, and you are preparing for what is to come. Decisions no longer stem from the intrapersonal conflict but rather from the freedom within your soul. The soul "lets loose" and enjoys freedom, basking in its liberty as an exhilarating feeling pours into the heart and mind.

Are you free or trapped in a restricted situation that refuses to change? Is there any potential in the situation identified? It is time to break bonds, bounds, and generational cycles of physical incapacitation and emotional and mental toxicity. A change ushers in a new era of personal growth, an age of the shining sun after the storm.

The question is, can you see the sun when it has yet to rise above the horizon? The journey to wellness has its ups and downs, and we know better than to seek to microwave the process. Since we know better, we should do better. A journey is like cooking a traditional Thanksgiving Dinner; we cannot microwave every dish and produce the desired meal. Though microwavable products are convenient, they also contain fillers and sodium, and they lack seasoning. If this is how you envision your ideal life, then let me know how that works out when you do not see the manifestation erect.

Journeys entail traveling from place to place, pacing the course, and learning along the way until milestones are achieved. The adventures are profound. They include experiences of landscapes, water bodies, and mountainous terrains. These serve as divine healing resources to help achieve wellness. These experiences and encounters, however challenging, afford moments of exultation. When I am running errands or traveling from one place to another, I often turn down the radio and take a few seconds to express my gratitude. For example, I often walk in front of the house to appreciate the outdoor environment— the birds, trees, flowers, and grass. I then watch the sunrise. There are times when I close my eyes and listen to the melody of the birds singing. I inhale fresh air and sweet fragrances of nature and exhale negativity and emotional toxins. Weekly, during the spring, summer, and fall, I walk barefoot across the grass to release muscle tensions and overcome stressors.

These are what we refer to as **S.M.A.R.T.** goals. They are *small, measurable, achievable, rational,* and *temporary (or time-bound).* Set attainable goals for yourself. Document your journey to wellness and track and celebrate each milestone, so you do not get lost in the process. Keep a record of turning points in your adventure; they serve as monuments both to appraise your progress and re-energize you in moments of forlorn anticipations and bleakness. You may need to ask for help—be it an experienced therapist, a tested-and-tried friend, a trustworthy family member, or a sound book. Or listen to soothing music. And very importantly, listen to your positive, hopeful inner voice—that "still, small voice" amid turmoil. Make it your compass to navigate over water, land, and air.

Pause, think, reflect, and reboot the self. If you stopped doing things you enjoyed because they have been trapped in a whirlwind of chaos, get out of your levity and superfluous frivolity and revisit those things that elevate you to the next level. This is the way to find your true purpose toward wellness. Break free of the chain of insecurities and test your limits. Be the sun— the conscious self-luminous heavenly body, constantly radiating happiness. Be the moon—the conscious satellite during eclipse and gloominess. Again, the objective is to enjoy the process and not to get lost in the storms. The journey is not about speed, for the moon has its own orbiting speed. It is not about immediate gratification, for there is time for everything under the sun. It is not about comparison, bragging rights, or testimonies, for each heavenly body has its own unique glory. It is about pacing, exploring, and enjoying life's journey to develop confidence in yourself more and more each day.

Journey to Wellness Self-Discovery Reflection

What intrapersonal battles are you constantly waging?

_____

_____

_____

_____

How do they affect the battles in your life?

_____

_____

_____

_____

How do you pacify these conflicts? With reactions or responses? Ignoring or suppressing?

_____

_____

_____

_____

Once you have identified your inner battles, how do you plan to rid yourself of them?

_____

_____

_____

_____

What steps to wellness will you take?

_____

_____

_____

_____

Do they involve self-reckoning and soul-searching?

_____

_____

_____

_____

Are you open to the process of change and growth?

_____

_____

_____

_____

Are you ready to embrace the driver's role seat in your life?

_____

_____

_____

_____

Set S.M.A.R.T Goals
Goals should be small, measurable, achievable, rational, and time-bound.

Track Progress
Document, journal, and record progress or lack thereof.

Self-Assess or Evaluate
Self-assess for patterns, successes, opportunities, and aspirations.

Ask for Help
Consider talking with a therapist or trustworthy loved-one.

Listen
Listen to soothing music, positive inner voice, or nothing at all.

In My Past Life

In the mirror of many an eye
I see my dead self-locked behind;
There animated in the lives of everyday people,
I see you when you are gone,
When you caved in into the womb of dusk
And dead silence sits on the throne
Where your voice is meant to thunder.
There in the stillness of the night
Stands your ghostly silhouette
Unmoving, helpless, forever.

I look upon your attire.
You are donned all over with forlorn
feeling of your epitaph
But knowing that this was me in the past,
before my rebirth,
Dear friend, I can empathize.

Reflecting on past experiences offers glimpses of who we were, but it also indicates who we are becoming. Once we are awakened and have emerged from the emotional dusk and puddles of tears, our third eye has gone through a partial soul development phase. We are quickened by unfamiliar and unprecedented strengths from a bloodline of tribal warriors and ancestors. Believe when I say, you are stronger than you think and more than a conqueror with extraordinary gifts. Jennifer Williams reminds us of that as she shares her intimate *Journey to Wellness* story of abuse, divorce, and loss. Lend your eyes and ears to Jennifer's journey as she advises we should listen more and talk less.

Emotional Wellness

Meet Jennifer Williams

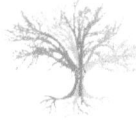

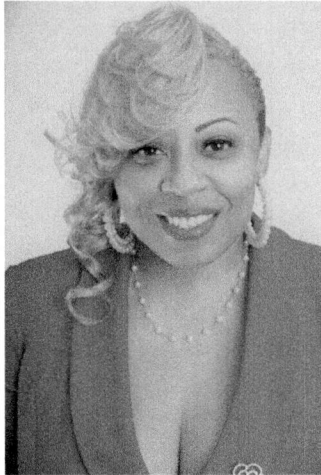

Proclaim:

Do not give up, even if you might be experiencing hell right now.
If you keep pushing through, greater awaits you on the other side.
You are not meant to lose the battle.

Introduction

Hi, my name is Jennifer Nicole Williams. Born in Gary, Indiana, on November 30, 1979, I am the oldest sibling on my family's side. My upbringing was somewhat normal. We lived with my grandmother most of the time until I was 21 years old, and then I finally moved out. Being a young and ambitious woman, I wanted to step into my own independence. I remember my grandmother being terribly upset about the move, so much so that she did not even say goodbye. She wanted me to stay longer, but it was time to gain my independence in this life. It was time to put into practice all I had learned from her as a young girl.

Shortly thereafter, at the age of 22, I became pregnant with my son, Micah, who is now 18 years old. Sweet Jesus, when my grandmother found out, she was livid. Although my son brings me tremendous joy, another child was not in my future unless it also accompanied a deep, secure, and loving marriage with my soulmate. After the birth of Micah, I saw life in a whole different light. In him, I found the motivation to make the most of my life and not just rest complacently in mediocrity. Even before his birth, I began to envision the life we deserve, and a part of the vision was homeownership. Though it took 11 years to accomplish that, I did it. My son took his first breath, and I changed for the better. I know so because I used to be a little reckless at times. I gave little or no thought at all to the consequences of my actions. For example, my temper often got the best of me. It altered my mood, displaying a concerning personality riddled with emotional dispositions and impulsive reactions. Sometimes all I saw was the color red, and I am not referring to romance. However, I was driven by this fiery passion. Many did not know my bad temper stemmed from the constant let-downs by people who vowed they absolutely loved me yet exhibited other intentions. Before I allowed my emotions to spiral out of control, I identified and understood what I was feeling and began to manage it by acknowledging and accepting them—all of them. It was important that I "not" transfer the hurt, pain, unproductive behaviors, and emotional reactions to Micah. He deserved so much more than my transgression. If I did not change, Micah would have been visiting his mother, not at her home, but in prison.

So, I turned my life around for the better. I would have loved to say it remained like so, but no, not precisely. I had many daunting challenges in life. Those challenges, however, were very instrumental in the making of the woman I am today. I went through an abusive relationship with my son's father that lasted for nine years. I walked away with the awareness of things I definitely did not want or deserve. But it took years of untold maltreatment to come to awareness and realize there was so much more than what that relationship was offering me. Nonetheless, I am grateful, not just for recovery from a traumatic relationship, but for everything I have endured the entire past 41 years. The unwavering verbal breaches and the struggle to keep my head up have nurtured inner power. I have done the work and earned every nickel, dime, and penny I possess.

I am immensely proud, not only for where I am today but also for where I am headed. It takes much grinding; yes, I know and have been at it for so long. I had been down to my last dime. I went through a really nasty divorce and allowed it to drive me to negative thinking for several months. But only those who quit finding themselves get stuck in quicksand. I considered my talents and available resources and turned those lemons into lemonade. It is through this "good" passion that I established three businesses from the ground up. Seeing how I was flourishing, I broadened my knowledge and sharpened my skill set to help people along the way.

After the divorce, many people noticed the awakening, and so did I. Now, I look at myself in the mirror and greet a refined, confident, and more fully realized African Goddess staring back at me. As funny as this statement may seem, but betrayal was a blessing. Everyone has a calling, and mine is to establish the foundation and pass the torch to the next generation before I exit this world.

Jennifer's Identified Trauma, Challenges, and Barriers
Abuse, Divorce, Loss, Relationship Trauma

Jennifer's Journey to Wellness Story
Wellness means you have made amends and now are at peace with yourself. My survival through difficult challenges was by getting closer to God. I mean, I wanted to be nowhere else. Who else wanted me? Where else am I accepted just as I am? I needed healing for myself and could not be found in the comfort of another man, alcohol, or substances. Even if there was a trace of it in them, I wanted none of those.

I buried myself in church. I was a walking mess for almost a year. My heart was shattered into so many pieces, and I needed help finding my way back to a healthy life, but not from man. First, I rededicated my life to God and let Him fully into my mind, body, and soul.

The healing process was not a cakewalk. I could not eat, sleep, or focus on anything, but the relationship hurt. I contemplated suicide because I could not withstand the pain. My face did not lack tears. My heart became familiar with achy palpitations. I cried every day for at least six months on end. Only family and a few close friends knew what I was enduring. Some made jokes, some laughed, and some even mocked me. A word to the wise, do not expect emotional support from those against the love or marriage you desire. They are anxiously listening for hiccups and waiting for failure so they can have the last word. "See? I knew it would not last." Know your adversaries as they enjoy "dumping" a bucket of salt on open wounds.

As I said, God was the only one to approach. Once I let God heal my heart, it was simply amazing. Not only does God mend the outside, He also heals you such that you are a completely different human on the inside as well. Anyone dealing with something excruciating in their personal life, I admonish you, allow God to heal you. I promise you will not regret it. I had to go through all I went through to come to the point of surrender, where God could steer my life in the way I ought to go. Yet even that recovery process is not without a cost. With God, all loss is not a loss! Keep that in mind when you are going through it.

Jennifer's Old Way of Thinking – Negative Thoughts

I suffered from low self-esteem. I think it was a consequence of the attitude of people I love towards me—people whose opinions and reactions I held in high esteem. I had gained 40 pounds during my marriage because I became complacent and nonchalant. My mate, in the end, did not want to touch me anymore. It felt like I disgusted him, which ate at me regularly. At a point, I felt utterly worthless. Although other people saw only my exterior and looked upon me as this strong, independent woman, on the inside, I was an insecure person who detested seeing herself in the mirror. A very disheartening experience it was.

Jennifer's Old Reactions and Behaviors

It was not how other people treated me that ate at me; rather, the attitude of one whom I took as my soulmate was the thing that gnawed at my very soul. The compliments stopped. The slaps on the butt ceased. The fire that was once there in his eyes was blown. The warmth perished. I remember one evening I desired his touch and sex. I reached for his body, but as soon as my hand touched him, he yelled, "Leave me the **** alone!" I was shocked. That reaction staggered me to my very roots. I could not believe what he said and the hateful look he gave. I could see the disgust in his eyes at that very moment. I cried myself to sleep. The person whom I was madly in love with was not in love with me. It was a hard pill to swallow, but evidently, the marriage was over. Physical affection was no longer my right to choose—a stark contrast to who he used to be. I recalled when I was more than enough. But now, suddenly, after four years, he could not stand my touch or the sound of my voice. Wow!

Because I am good at concealing pain, no one knew I was dying on the inside. You have to be close to me before you could suspect when something is troubling me. It is an awful habit, but I mask the pain until I shatter into pieces. I will hold it in, and no one would suspect when something is upsetting me. At first, I did not notice I could be such a tough cookie. Perhaps this is because it was settled knowledge that people tend to take advantage of me when my cards are shown. So, while people thought I was doing fine in my marriage, I was a complete mess.

Jennifer's New Way of Thinking – Positive Thoughts

"I can do all things through Christ who strengthens me." When you think negatively, you attract bad things to manifestation in your life. So, I speak positively and move positively. Being upset takes too much work and energy. I love to smile and maintain a positive space and atmosphere. See the good in all things.

Jennifer's New Responses and Behaviors

I fix my thoughts on God's blessings. I look at how God has blessed me despite the major setbacks I have endured in life.

27

Unwanted events do occur, but I choose to see good in everything.

I lost my job nine months ago. My boss, who I thought of as more than just my boss, reported me. How come? They complained that my business constituted a conflict of interest in the company because she assumed I was conducting personal business at work. My then boss called human resources (HR) and reported the concern. Not given any notice or a hearing, I was accused and fired before they confirmed the allegations. When she barged into my office questioning the client, he told her I completed his taxes over the weekend at home. (I helped so many people with the knowledge I had accumulated over the years from previous jobs or knowledge acquired through research.) She then looked puzzled, and her face turned red. However, she had already reported the accusations to HR before confirming the rumor. The very next day, without even a conversation from HR, I was terminated—such a reward for three years of diligent service. I had no documented write-ups, only impressive branch sales, and outstanding performance evaluations, and I only called off once in three years. Just like that, I was deleted. But not once did I worry because if God could ordain something so small, He can also provide something much more significant than that job.

The funny thing is, within 24 hours of the termination, my commercial loan was approved to purchase a building for my tax and credit repair business. I never mourned the job loss because I invested my energy into celebrating the new venture. You see, what they meant for evil, God turned it around to work out in my favor. I remember exiting the building, and the regional manager looked and said, "Call me if you need something." I looked that woman squarely in her eyes and said, confidently, "I won't be needing anything from you." I walked out of the building with my head held high!

It was time to close a chapter with an establishment that did not acknowledge my worth. No, they were too blinded with envy even to see it. When people see you being elevated, they view you as a threat. You remember the saying, "You can do good but not as good as or better than me!" Since I left the nine-to-five job, it has only been blessings on top of blessings. Getting terminated was a blessing in disguise. You see, I have no time to think negatively. Every time something seemingly negative happens, it is replaced with a blessing. This is how I know God is making room for more extraordinary things and removing old things from my life. I am grateful for the journey to wellness. There have been highs and lows, but I simply let God's plan for my life prevail. If you trust the process, you will get all God has ordained for your life. No one ever said the process would be easy, but it is worth what you went through.

While pacing through the healing process, I emerged a different woman. I reached a point where I had no desire to entertain the old me. Transformed into a beautiful creature on the inside and out, my thirst for life had changed for the better. And now, some cannot handle the new and improved me. Things that used to matter are now simply things of the past. I am in such a good place in life that it sometimes feels surreal. I look myself in the mirror from time to time and ask, "Who are you, girl?" I cannot believe how far I have come in two years and counting.

Jennifer's Restoration Tip

It was simple. You either sink or swim. I have never been a quitter, so sinking was not among the options. In addition to that, I had a child who was silently observing. I chose to show him that even though there are setbacks in life, do not just lie there in the failure and waste away. The unspoken mentorship I promised my son eventually motivated me. Because I knew he was watching, I had to pull it together. I looked hard at self and desired to succeed. I believe this is also applicable to everyone: we all have someone, if not a multitude, whose life achievements depend on whether we fail or succeed. We may not know them yet, but God has ordained it so. I desire to leave this earth as one of the most influential women in the world. So, there is much work to do. This is the goal that gives me the motivation and enthusiasm to succeed.

Jennifer's Definition of Success

Success is a continuous grind to the finish line. If you keep moving, treat people right, then producing is inevitable. God will give you the desires of your heart. This is my approach to success. Remember, somebody is always watching. The right people will be put in your path to assist you in getting to the next level. Keep grinding!

Jennifer's Journey to Wellness Takeaway

One of the vital lessons I have garnered, especially in relationships with people, is *never to move too fast*. First, analyze the whole situation. Do not be so much in a rush to do things. Anything that comes too fast is dangerous. Pay close attention to those red flags because if you do not, you will pay severely in the end.

Jennifer Advises

The best advice is to listen more and talk less. People will tend to tell on themselves. Listen for inconsistencies. If someone is rushing into doing something, always know there is a hidden agenda. Always pray for discernment when dealing with anything or anyone you are unsure of. Never avoid red flags. If something seems too good to be true, trust your gut!

Journey to Wellness Practical Tool

Cognitive – Old Way of Thinking - Negative Thoughts
Instructions: Pause and take three deep breaths to clear the mind, then complete the exercise. List three negative self-thoughts you experienced during this chapter.

_____

_____

_____

_____

Emotional – Accepting Feelings and Emotions – Negative or Positive
Instructions: Pause and take three minutes to notice and connect with your feelings, then complete the exercise. Identify, list, and recite three emotions you are feeling at a particular moment. Be compassionate with yourself.

_____

_____

_____

_____

Cognitive, Emotional, and Behavioral – New Way of Thinking, Responses, and Behaviors
Instructions: Reflect on the questions throughout the chapter, explore new thoughts and desired changes. Rewrite the three negative thoughts listed above into positive thoughts.

_____

_____

_____

_____

Recite each rewritten positive thought three different times throughout the day. Remember to use a compassionate tone. Journal the times below.

_____

_____

_____

_____

Name three adjectives to describe how you felt after the positive self-talk exercise.

_____

_____

_____

_____

List three ways how you will think or respond differently to adverse challenges in the future.

_____

_____

_____

_____

PART TWO

Understanding Evidence-Based Approaches

Though the book is based on personal experiences, I also desire to offer and bring awareness to evidence-based approaches and tools to encourage, inspire, and motivate readers across the world who may not be familiar with these options. Cognitive-Behavioral Therapy and Positive Psychology are evidence-based therapeutic options that are effective and applicable to address a wide range of problems.

Cognitive-Behavioral Therapy

Cognitive-behavioral therapy (CBT) was born around the 1980s by combining two emerging approaches in psychology: behavioral and cognitive psychology. Unlike other psychotherapeutic approaches, such as the psychoanalytic approach, CBT focuses on "problem-solving." Therapists and clinicians help the patient search for the best strategies to change and reduce distress symptoms. It also focuses on changing one's negative default thoughts that contribute to emotional difficulties, depression, and anxiety.

CBT allows you to gradually face a series of anxious circumstances, starting from the least demanding to the most complex ones. Little by little, the patient relearns to manage previously avoided situations and/or evoked negative thoughts. CBT aims not simply to eliminate negative thoughts but to know how to manage them concretely by modifying emotions, behaviors, and dysfunctional thoughts. Therefore, the treatment aims to improve patients 'quality of life and help them manage or resolve any psychopathology. CBT provides the tools to identify distorted patterns of reasoning and interpretation of reality, then integrates them with functional and positive thoughts and beliefs.

Principles of Cognitive Behavioral Therapy

In the cognitive-behavioral approach, the classic cognitive treatment (i.e., the analysis and refutation of dysfunctional thoughts) remains central and, as mentioned previously, is integrated by the contributions of behaviorism and functional analysis.

In fact, in cognitive-behavioral psychotherapy, thoughts, emotions, and behaviors influence each other. Negative dysfunctional thoughts such as "nobody likes me" or "I am an unpleasant person" can lead the person to feel sadder or more discouraged (negative emotions) and lead them to reduce the opportunities for socializing and shut themselves up at home (dysfunctional behavior).

Similarly, behaviors also influence thoughts and emotions. For example, isolation and closeness in the house (dysfunctional behaviors) can reinforce the thought "nobody likes me" because it cannot be refuted by experience (leaving the house, one might find that someone likes me). Furthermore, isolation reduces social relationships, and pleasant activities carried out daily, thus favoring the emergence of feelings of sadness and reinforcing dysfunctional thoughts.

Techniques in Cognitive Behavioral Therapy

Over the years, different psychotherapeutic techniques have been studied. In the context of CBT, the main techniques are:

- Self-instruction (e.g., conscious use of distraction techniques or positive self-talk);
- Relaxation or biofeedback techniques
- Identification and refutation of negative thoughts
- Home exercises or live exhibitions
- Imaginative displays
- Mindfulness exercises
- Skills training

Positive Psychology

Positive Psychology is a movement within the psychological sciences in the 1990s. The movement emphasizes the role of the individual's potential and resources in terms of acceptance, adaptation, courage, action, awareness, creativity, flexibility, and responsibility.

Everyone's life has peaks and valleys, and positive psychology in no way denies human suffering. Its premise is more balanced: what is good in life is equally genuine as what is bad and therefore deserves equal attention from psychologists. Thus, positive psychology starts with the idea that life involves more than avoiding or solving problems. It is a psychological approach which studies, scientifically, how to promote the strengths and virtues of the human character, such as optimism, joy, inspiration, motivation, and a sense of humor, among others, to be able to develop and enhance a positive attitude to live a full, fluid life and as a prevention of mental health pathologies.

Positive Psychology is one of the most recent trends in psychology that focuses on the study of experiences and positive traits. It studies the strengths, virtues, motivations, and capacities of individuals and how these characteristics help improve their quality of life and enhance their personal development. Usually, the different psychological theories have focused on explaining and studying the different mental pathologies and individuals' negative behaviors. However, Positive Psychology explores strategies to achieve and optimize our personal strengths. It focuses attention on the prevention of different mental problems.

The Purpose of Positive Psychology

For a long time, psychology has focused on the pathological, on the negative, from which all the aspects of problem-solving we already know have arisen. In this way, this approach can open doors to a new way of thinking to discover everything positive within, which makes us happy and excited to achieve a greater outlook on life. Therefore, the ultimate goal of positive psychology is to identify and enhance strengths (prevention and preservation) to cultivate personal talents toward a sense of optimism.

The way reality is interpreted changes the experience of reality itself, and the more one does it through positive emotions, the more one can grow from it. Focusing more on what is negative predisposes you to stress and anxiety while bringing your mind to a state of positivity allows you to improve your performance, become more solid, and better face the challenges that life inevitably presents.

Positive Psychology Exercises

Practice Gratitude

Gratitude is probably one of the most well-known positive psychology exercises. It involves focusing on the present moment and appreciating what is rather than what could or should be. Those who practice gratitude regularly experience more positive emotions, feel more alive, and show more empathy. They also benefit from a more robust immune system.

Gratitude Letter Writing (or Gratitude Visit)

Think of a person who played a significant (positive) role in your life but whom you never thanked properly. Write a letter in which you describe in detail what they did and the impact they had on you. Be specific and let go (You will have an opportunity to read an example and complete this exercise later on in Part Three titled *Dear Black Man*).

Three Good Things

Before going to bed, write down three things you enjoyed on this day. Then explain the "why" behind the good. Think about the impact these events had and how the day would have been if they had not happened. For example, I had an excellent date with Terrence last night. Why? Because we had a meaningful conversation, and he shared three things he loved about me. Make a habit of writing and celebrating positive things that have happened every day.

Smile

Smile because you can! A killer smile is a formidable weapon to feel good. Simply activating specific facial muscles can turn our mood from negative to positive, and the impact on others can be significant. Take this test: when you meet someone, be the first to smile and observe the results. The power of such a simple action is impressive.

Visualize Success

Visualizing the road to success creates a mental image that builds self-confidence. To do this, find a quiet place to sit, close your eyes, and relax. Visualize yourself completing a task successfully. These exercises help relax the body and mind. They create a feeling of calm and well-being that strengthens your focus and decreases stress. If you have a hard time visualizing success or just want to try something different, picture the desired state of mind, such as relaxation, contentment, or peace. Imagine a comfortable, pleasant place, a location you associate with the mood you desire and do so by imagining every detail and using all five known senses. For example, if you are walking in a forest, notice the wind on your back, birds chirping, and the smell of flowers permeating the air. You will also notice a shift in focus, muscles relaxing, deep breathing, and feeling a deep sense of peace, appreciation, and contentment. Such visualization is a staycation for the mind.

Practice Self-Compassion

We all tend to be hard on ourselves, each to varying degrees. We are critical and find fault with the slightest imperfection. By correcting and amplifying our mistakes and faults, we get into the habit of focusing on the negative. Not only does this damage our self-esteem and self-confidence, but it also shifts our mood. It impairs our ability to experience positive experiences and events in our lives fully. Remember, self-compassion is the natural antidote to perfectionism and self-criticism through the benevolent recognition of our imperfections.

Reverse Focus

Most people tend to dwell on the negative rather than the positive emotions or aspects of an event. Reverse the focus and shift the attention to more positive aspects of life. I use this technique when I am socializing in negative group settings where individuals focus on hypotheticals instead of the facts. You can also use this technique to reflect on the day before bedtime. Think about what went well and journal the why. Another method is compiling a list of daily accomplishments and expressing self-gratitude.

Feed Hope

One way to cultivate hope is to reduce the scale of the problem—perhaps by breaking the problem down into smaller pieces to address or accomplish over time. Another way is to identify the healthy, positive skills and coping mechanisms to help overcome the challenge and then develop a measurable, realistic, obtainable plan.

Mindfulness Meditation

Mindfulness meditation focuses on the present moment. It involves paying attention to our thoughts without judgment and with kindness. Instead of focusing on what we should be feeling, it assists with being aware of what we are actually feeling at the very moment. It is not about a modification but connecting to the here-and-now experience. What matters is "what is" versus "what should be."

These exercises are tools that can easily be incorporated into daily activities. Choose one or two mindfulness meditation exercises that resonate with your heart and soul and execute. Like the gym, start by practicing the exercises three times a week for ten to 30 minutes a day and increase and deepen the practice as you master your skills. There is no rush. On a basic level, pacing helps release the notion of limited time, tension, and stress. It is also a reminder to enjoy the moment and embrace your creative potential because it is limitless. Creativity is like my grandma turning leftovers into a meal to feed all nine of her grandchildren. It is the smarts and heart to make something unique you will not find on Winn-Dixie, Kroger, or Publix grocery store shelves. Although she did not have much money, she found a way to ensure that her grandchildren were fed. Creativity will make a way out of no way. Some say it is God; I say it is the God in you.

Pacing Strides

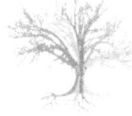

Proclaim:

*I AM pacing my stride
with a smile and embracing
the steps to learn and heal.*

Whether you like it or not, taking shortcuts only takes you right back to square one. I am here to forewarn you to stay far away from taking shortcuts. It is an alluring trap that appears to look and feel appealing in the interim, but the long-term effects might take a lifetime to rectify its grave mistake. Moreover, it creates roadblocks by circumventing the preparation stages necessary to obtain the very thing you desire.

I cannot think of any worthwhile venture that does not have a process. There is none, is there? The purpose of having a process is similar to why many organizations adopt *Robert's Rules of Order.* It offers structure and consistency. There is Step 1, Step 2, Step 3, Step 4, and so forth. The process describes the "how" and the "why." Together, they provide a road map to maintain focus on improving the "how" and leaving it open to suggestions and modifications if one or more steps do not produce desired goals or expected outcomes. And, if you so choose to deviate from this set process, you are officially out of compliance even if you skip one step. Consider the process aborted.

Primary example: my nephew and I had season passes to Six Flags in Georgia for years. Being between the ages of three and five and the only child, patience was not his virtue. As a parental figure, duty rested on me to inculcate virtue to him. And I tell you, there were moments where I felt like pulling the hair out my beard. There were many instances when we stood in line, sometimes for more than an hour, to get on a single ride. Parents and caregivers, you know exactly what I am talking about. Any advertised ride on the cartoon channel instantly became the thing to do, a must-ride for our children. This is where I slapped my forehead. But you know, we will do anything for the kids.

Because I loved him so much, I sought to avoid long lines. I thought it would be a good idea to purchase flash passes until I saw the prices. Though my love ran deep, my pockets did not, and we ended up standing in long lines instead, suntanning all summer by force. It was fine with me; they say the blacker the berry, the sweeter the juice. Well I was one "ole" sweet, tasty fruit snack for someone to eat. In essence, I am saying that it was frustrating for him; for me, it was saving money—not to mention I did not mind the wait. So, what did I choose to do? I kindly turned it into a learning activity. This allowed him to demonstrate and master the process of patience. Over the years, time after time, we stood in long lines waiting for our turn to enjoy the rides he picked. Sometimes he found himself skipping lines as if he were an adolescent Black Superman. When it happened, I approached him gingerly, grabbed his hand, and escorted him back to his appropriate place in line.

Here is my opportunity to be a model uncle. I pulled him aside and explained the process. Parents, you know how the moral talk goes. At the age of three, he gave me a confused look but finally said, "Okay." What other choice did he have? To reaffirm the principle and be sure he understood, I asked, "Nephew, do you understand what I am saying?" He responded, "Yes, I understand." Did he like the talk? Probably not. However, this was the park's process, and these were the park rules. And anyone who would be truly successful and well in life should better learn this from childhood. Life teaches us that organizations have guidelines, policies, and procedures in order to increase revenue and assets and decrease expenditures and other liabilities. Consider applying similar processes during your journey to wellness. Have you labeled your journey stages as assets or liabilities? There is a difference. And the process—or shortcut, as the case may be—makes the difference.

There are many circumstances in which we would like to take the short route. Why not defy the 65 or 70 miles per hour speed limit on interstate highways when the car's speed goes up to 130 miles per hour? Why not defy the parking lot's rule as indicated by the white arrows when you can drive directly through it when it is not so crowded? As simple as these regulations may seem, they can have grave consequences. A primary reason these road laws and practices are in place is to prevent harm. Driving 30 miles per hour is too slow; it will take you forever to reach the location, and it will impede traffic. Driving 95 miles per hour is too fast and will make it difficult to break timely if needed to and you may potentially receive a super speeder ticket, not to mention a suspended driver's license. However, pacing the drive at 65 or 70 miles per hour (plus or minus ten miles per hour) decreases the chances of receiving a ticket or causing an accident. Yet, you would arrive at the destination at an appropriate time. Structures exist to promote a steady rhythm, a cadence, a pace that ensures decorum, decency, and consistency. Therefore, avoid extremes, or you will eventually stall and drift into a rut. Do not be so obsessed with the end results that you missed the details of your breakthrough.

Be patient and improve your function and perform steadily, "one mile per hour" like you are coasting the highway.

It may just be your "luck" if while driving through the parking lot and not follow the arrows, out of nowhere, a car appears and strikes you, causing damages all on account of failure to adhere to the instructional directions, otherwise known as the process. Shortcuts are deadly, believe me, and they never turn into the good success you have hoped for. Back alleys and back doors may get you to a location faster, but the long-term reality turns out quite differently. Your destination becomes uncertain, and you find yourself amidst a myriad of other troubles and worries.

The journey to wellness is also a process. I recommend learning how to make it enjoyable, manageable, and obtainable. Nowadays, we tend to believe and buy into other systems and processes, hoping to see a quick turnaround. Remember that someone else's journey, however, is not your journey; therefore, the odds of a quick turnaround while operating in someone else's system are likely not with you. Take this truth from me—been there, done that.

When you have chosen the authentic route, at times, you will find it to be exhausting and even frustrating. As these moments show up, and they will, use the proposed techniques provided in the book; it will help decrease stress and anxiety so you can step back, survey the situation, and move forward with a logical plan of resolve. Approach it from a third-person perspective. We can usually offer advice to other people on their matters of urgency and distress, but we are often left entirely clueless when it comes to issues in our own lives. This is so because we are usually not as emotionally invested in other people's situations or circumstances, so we can remain somewhat neutral and observe the situation from a wise viewpoint where the cacophony of the situation would not interfere with your decision-making. However, when we need to shift the spotlight on ourselves and assess the circumstance, here are a few rules to assist with our own journey to wellness.

Three Rules to Assist Your Journey to Wellness

First and foremost, we must dispel marketing tactics that suggest achieving results can happen in the blink of an eye. Even the lottery has its odds. What is preventing you from enjoying your wellness journey? Is it that you have bought into someone else's process? Let us consider nutritional health as an example. Did you know that most of the food commercials on television are loaded with carbohydrates and sugars, in other words, often misleading and delivering false promises? Take a closer look at their marketing labels and what demographic population in which they are marketing. I am not advising you against any product. However, I recommend that you understand the product and the system that makes millions off your hard-earned dollar. Additionally, I encourage people to invest in the stocks of the company from which they purchase products. That means if you buy groceries from Walmart or fill prescriptions at Walgreens, then every paycheck, take $0.50 up to $100, if you can afford it, and invest in that company. Why not financially benefit from companies that are financially benefiting from you?

Every two weeks, I invest small amounts of money, automatically deducted from my banking account, into General Mills. Why? Because my nephew loves cereal. Have you seen the cereal prices these days? They are $4 to $5 a box. Let me push pause on this financial topic and return to the original discussion. However, I felt the need to drop a golden nugget or two at your doorstep. But before we move on, let us partake in this exercise and speak abundance into our lives.

*Grab your wallet, place it in the palm of your hand, and cover it fully with the other hand. Take deep breaths and hold it for three seconds. Now recite, "**My actions attract more abundance into my life**." Repeat the process two more times, then exhale.*

I speak financial wellness into your life; you, too, should do so. Now, back to the three rules to assist your journey to wellness.

Rule #1 - Facts are Facts

Everything that looks, sounds, and tastes good does not always mean it is good for you. To achieve nutritional wellness goals, the first rule of thumb is reading all labels and related information. Walk into any grocery store as a consumer, and you run directly into marketing and advertisements. Before we read what is in the box, we look at what is on the front of it and overlook the written information on the side. Ignore the pretty packaging and fancy, highlighted fonts, and move directly to what some refer to as the boring black and white nutritional content label. When shopping for cereal, milk, or juice, always read the nutritional label first; they highlight the facts. According to the U.S. Food and Drug Administration, they require nutritional label updates, including scientific information, new nutrition research, and public information changes. That is huge. We can see exactly what we are digesting.

Although the Federal Trade Commission (FTC) Act prohibits unfair or deceptive advertising, companies still find creative strategies that are quite misleading to increase their profit margin by persuading consumers to believe and buy into their persuasion. The FTC states that advertising must tell the truth and not mislead consumers. But understand that advertising and marketing are never just advertising and marketing—they are sprinkled with several untruths. After reading nutritional labels, look at the marketing image, and ask yourself if it is indeed a representative of you or who you are striving to become. Suppose you do not know who you are and for what you are aiming for. In that case, the label interpretations may lead to unhealthy or harmful thinking, such as feeling you are not beautiful because your body is shaped disproportionately and not like the image on the package. Before you know it, you have grabbed and purchased the product just because the messaging suggests it will fix the issue. Have you had these thoughts before? How many products have you purchased due to an emotional reaction and later realized it was not the best decision? Next time, before purchasing a product, first read the label. Then, look at the image and ask if it represents your journey. Last, ask yourself, "How does it emotionally affect me?" These challenging questions will help process the situations more clearly so you can respond, not react, to them more effectively. Avoid being persuaded by marketing illusions, as they distract the eye from reality and modify the truth, whereas labels state the facts.

In my past life, I lived to eat. But since my chronic kidney disease diagnosis in 2012, I adopted a new mantra. Right now, *I eat to live* (as living to eat). What does that mean? It means I spend ample time understanding what I consume before consuming it instead of continuing the old habit of eating carelessly. Do not get me wrong, I respect and love all the foodies across the globe, and I love to eat like the next person. But if you aim to eat to live, it is easy to see that you just cannot consume everything that satisfies your taste buds the way you want. In conversing with a friend, he was adamant about hiring a personal trainer to shed a few pounds. My response was, "If losing weight is the goal, then focus on your nutritional intake instead of hiring a personal trainer, and you will achieve the results you desire." Although I provided an appropriate response, I should have said, "If you change the mind and change the food, then the goal will follow." However, that is not how the conversation developed. I explained that nutrition is far more important than exercise when it comes to losing weight. Focus on consuming recommended calculated macros intended for your weight, and the calorie deficit will follow. Unfortunately, after the back and forth, and he did not absorb the information offered. To my readers, if you are considering hiring a personal trainer but are having a difficult time managing nutrition, there is a high probability that you will not optimize the results desired. Again, change the thoughts (cognitive); the thoughts will change nutritional intake (behavior), and then proper nutrition will change the body (physical).

Reading food labels can look foreign to beginners. I suggest finding a reputable research-based website or magazine that explains the scientific terms and information on everything listed on nutrition labels. Until you can complete the research, here is a quick note to get you started. Run to the kitchen and grab a food box and look at the ingredient list at the bottom. The ingredients are listed in order, from the greatest used amount first, followed in descending order of ingredients until the smaller amount is reached. For instance, if the first ingredient is fructose, you are consuming simple sugar, which makes up to roughly 50% of table sugar known as sucrose. If the goal is to decrease calories, then this is an ingredient you must reduce. Always read the labels because the facts are the facts.

Rule #2 - Know Your Strengths and Weaknesses

Next is knowing your strengths and weaknesses. Everything in life has an opposite. For us to appreciate one, we have to understand or experience the other. For example: sad and happy, safety and danger, salt and sugar, scream and whisper, and satisfaction and regret. To appreciate strengths or weaknesses, we have to identify and understand their value. One of the most powerful ways to transform one's life is by identifying, understanding, and knowing strengths and weaknesses. This enables you to determine when to step-up and step-out and when to step back, shut up, listen, and observe.

Our strengths and weaknesses are functions of our talents, skills, and abilities, which vary from person to person. Some skills are intrinsic, and some are learned and developed over time. The beauty of strengths and weaknesses is that they foster collaborations and birth valuable relationships, new energy, fresh vision, and purposeful living. Collaboration enables us to work together by sharing passions, ideas, and visions to achieve a common, defined purpose for our partners and stakeholders.

Many believe it is risky to discuss or show weakness. That is both true and untrue. If someone on the team has ill or malicious intentions, then it holds true; you are very well at a high risk of being hoodwinked. However, if team members are each other's keepers and watch each other's back, we are at minimum risk or no risk bearing our strengths and weaknesses. Such a team is committed to teaching and training can view mistakes as growth opportunities to develop each member. By being observant, meticulous, and modeling after great exemplars, you will experience incremental changes in your strength while overcoming weaknesses over time.

A decade-plus years ago, I attended a leadership conference. The CEO opened the meeting with an inspiring speech. He had to have been about 57 years old, standing 5'9, weighing 193 pounds, Caucasian, white-haired, round face with glasses, and a voice that projected into the hall. He mentioned that as a child, he stuttered frequently and significantly. His speech was choppy, and he had a difficult time saying what he thought or felt. His mother, bent on helping him conquer his speech impediment (weakness), enrolled him in speech therapy (resource/opportunity). Over time, the teachings and training strengthened his speech, which also boosted his confidence and self-esteem. He turned a noticeable weakness into a remarkable strength because someone identified his weakness and saw potential growth.

Our minds are so conditioned that most times when we hear the word "weakness," we start to define it in terms of "less than" or "lack of." For me, weakness stands for a call and privilege to develop a technique or skill that I have yet to acquire or master. And while I am doing so, I am to use my already existing strengths to compensate for weaknesses, help balance emotional upsets, provide safety and security, and volunteer them to assist in developing others who are experiencing weaknesses in areas I am not. Part of our journey is to serve. If your schedule allows even 15 to 30 minutes two to three times a week, consider allocating time to mentor *Burgeoning Souls*, who shall eventually carry the legacy you established. Personal growth happens when we are consciously aware of our strengths and weaknesses. Be aware. Learn always. Be ever-evolving and ever-changing.

Rule #3 - Be Persistent but Pace Yourself

Here is a scenario: I planned a hiking trip. We were headed to the North Georgia Mountains. "Let's be adventurous," I said. "Pack your bags into the bus, and we are going to bond with nature. Oh, and by the way, I did not rent a cabin or reserve a hotel, so be prepared to remain persistent in facing your fears in the natural elements." That last piece of advice was for everyone to be thoughtful and purposeful when packing. That included considering appropriate clothing, shoes, accessories, and how much to grab because the trip required everyone to carry their own baggage. Things to consider were heat, rain, cold, and wildlife we may encounter. Mobile devices were restricted to everyone except me for safety purposes.

Imagine joining this retreat in the wooded mountains without paved roads, no outside distractions, critters roaming the

51

land, encroaching high elevated mountain peaks, and sleeping in the wild the entire weekend. Each day of persistent change is the soul seeking solutions to reduce unwanted static interference towards success. This is what I refer to as soul development.

Honestly, I am not sure how I would respond to an outdoor camping retreat as much as I love nature. Maybe I will book a wellness cabin retreat one year, then a wellness outdoor camping retreat the following year. Maybe. How does that sound to you? Let me know @*lovespursuitatl*.

The scenario I have just painted sounds like another season of the reality show "Survivor." The only difference is you are not competing against anyone else except for the inner self and its baggage. Think about the many emotions that will surge through your whole being for isolating from everyday activities, placed in an unfamiliar area, with unfamiliar people, and plunged into strange, unusual circumstances. Well, our journey to wellness is quite similar. There is a gradual transition from one lifestyle to another by persevering through survival skills despite opposition.

Some people are gifted with the ability to make an instantaneous change. Others are not; it must be gradual, beginning with the least task. I have encountered individuals who woke up in the emergency room to severe medical conditions due to an abrupt change in their circumstances. There was no notice, no warning, or no alarm.

If you are reading this book, that means there is a trace of hope in your soul. Really quickly, place your dominant hand on your chest. Inhale and exhale slowly. Repeat and pace the breathing. Now feel and watch your diaphragm contract as it moves up and down. When you breathe, it increases the chest cavity space, and the lungs expand, filling that area. Your journey is very similar; there are ups and downs, but it can lead to expansion. So, if you can breathe, then you can expand, and expansion results in a change.

Gradual change, consistency, vigilance, and persistence can sustain the determination to achieve success. The oppositions and harsh conditions will test your determination. It is where the rubber meets the road and the moment of truth. If the goal is to expand and extend your life expectancy and fulfill life's purpose, pace the journey, and push through the elements that beset you. Prepare well and arm yourself with all necessary apparatus. But if for some reason you are deficient in any of the required devices (in other words, you have a peculiar weakness), do not beat yourself up nor suddenly give up, for there must be someone in your "tribe" to succor you.

Moreover, you are not alone. There is a person in front of you, behind you, and on both sides of you for support when running low on food, energy, water, or heat. When you feel like you are running out of breath and your muscles are beginning to fatigue, help is not far away. Every one of us has vowed to reach out and grab your hand to pull you up or whisper a motivational word into your ear, "You got this." The journey may appear rougher than envisaged or longer than measured, but with like-minded souls around you and a clear, concise plan, it makes the journey much less stressful and worthwhile exploring. Do not give up. Remember to **Read the Facts**, **Know Your Strengths and Weaknesses**, and **Be Persistent** but **Pace the Journey**.

Three Rules to Assist Your Journey to Wellness

Facts are Facts
Take time to read and enjoy things that matter most.

Know Your Strengths and Weakness
Strengths and weaknesses are collaboration codes words for
opportunities.

Be Persistent, but Pace Yourself
There is no need to rush. Your time is your time.

Journey to Wellness Self-Discovery Reflection

What has prevented you in the past from being consistent?

_____
_____
_____
_____

What are the distractions in your life that forced you to ditch the process? Have you ever taken shortcuts?

_____
_____
_____
_____

How did they prove detrimental to your process?

_____
_____
_____
_____

What are your strengths and weaknesses? Try to incorporate family and friends to help with this exercise.

_____
_____
_____
_____

How can you develop your weaknesses with the help of your strengths?

_____
_____
_____
_____

You Are What You Eat!

If you are eating in order to live,
Why do you die from eating?
If you over speed to beat the traffic,
Why held down by the sheriff?
If you jump the line just to beat the time,
Cuffs and cells could be your fine.
What is your accomplishment and gain?
When your loss surpasses your strain?
In spite of all, you spend on coaches and gym,
You're worse off by what you feed.
Much is flowing into your big bucket
But the bottom is a basket!
Stop and reconsider
And think through your answer:
If you are eating in order to live,
Why do you die from eating?

Happiness is not a destination. We have lived and are living convoluted lives for most of us, and pacing our journey will support modest steps toward modest victories. Note that happiness is not directional and does not come with an instruction manual. It is a state of mind that chips away at old hurts, thoughts of loss and lost, and a bucketful of confusion. Sometimes most of our confusion is from a lack of focus, creative expression, and nutrition. What and how are you feeding your creative space? Many are not aware that creative nutrition is just as crucial as food nutrition and physical exercise. Rashad Terry, a trained dancer, and skincare and make-up expert shares the dark side of creative expression. He spotlights creativity, love, and passion, and how love and passion drained his creativity dry until he met purpose. You see, love and passion can also chip away at your happiness. If you continue to buy into the idea that you should do what you love without purpose, burnout will soon follow. However, when purpose marries love and passion, you will value your gifts and actively participate in a diverse range of self-voyages. It means you are understanding and appreciating all parts of you with a high value.

Creative Wellness

Meet Rashad Terry

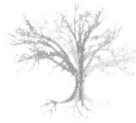

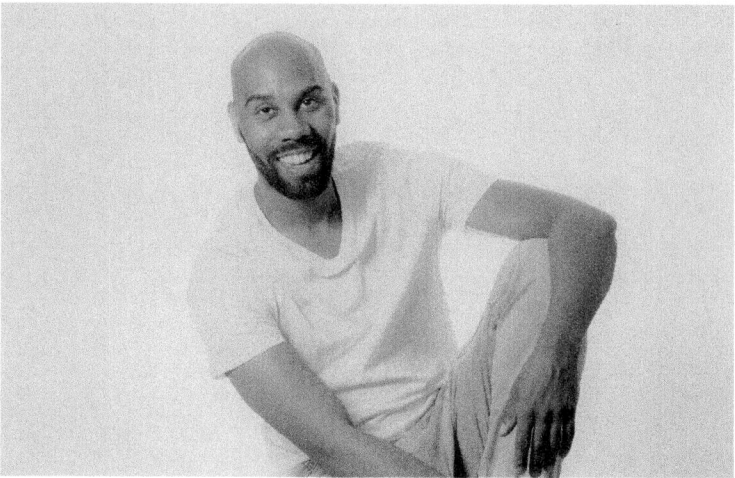

Proclaim:

I am a miraculous, amazing, worthy, confident human being,
and I am being led by the Spirit of God.
Everything I do is successful because I put the work in for it.

58

I am Powerful, Wealthy, Smart, Accomplished, and
Successful.
I am financially stable enough to truly afford the
things that I desire,
and not just what my budget limits me to.

I am happy within myself first,
I am manifesting a confident mindset,
I am stress-free,
I am depression-free,
I am living in what I desire,
I am Beautiful,
I am Stunning,
I am physically fit,
My health is at its best.

Introduction

Hi, my name is Rashad. I was born and raised in Miami, Florida, and grew up in a loving, kind, and gentle home with my three siblings, mother, and stepfather. Although my biological father did not raise me, our household, particularly myself, did not lack the example of a male figure. He excelled above every other bona fide father, any time, any day. My father taught me everything from changing brakes on a car to replacing drywall and cooking dinner. My parents were very attentive and involved. However, of the four of us, I was always the "quiet one," not very social at all. As a matter of fact, the only time I talked was when around my siblings and close friends. To an extent, I am still like that to this day. Well, unless someone places makeup, a couple of makeup brushes, and skincare products at my doorstep. Then, I become Puff the Magic Dragon or Jem from the Holograms: the spirit of creativity, amour, freedom, fun, and support.

All I knew as a child was dance. I lived and breathed it as a repertory company member for United Dancers of Miami. I also attended The Miami Conservatory for Ballet and danced for The Miami Cultural Arts Center for extra classes when I had the chance. I just knew my life would lead me to a long career in dance.

Dance pretty much consumed my life from middle school all through college. I attended The New World School of Arts for college. After that, I opened a dance studio and danced in several companies in Miami, also teaching. I created a pretty decent life for myself through dance. But it was not to be sustained because the deeper I dove into dance as a career, the more the business side of it sucked the passion out. I got to a point where the thing I once loved was misused and became an instrument of abuse by others against me, so much so that I lost the passion for it. Little did I know that passion is not as important as purpose; it was not long before I learned that purpose fuels passion. The purpose is actually the gas that drives life's journey to fulfillment.

So, I found a new interest and ventured into the beauty industry, learning everything I could. I went to Beauty Schools of America for Hair and Makeup, Academy of Glam for Makeup, and Aveda for Esthetics. It became addictive, almost as alluring as dance. I thought to myself, could this be true? Is it possible that I might have found a match, if not a substitute, which is similar to the feelings when I pirouette? Well, at least, I thought? The time and energy I poured into lifts, kicks, and spins were gradually transferred to textures, colors, and sheens. This is it; my creative mind eventually connected and aligned with the emotional and spiritual parts of me.

It was then I knew life was bigger than dance, so I now understand that dancing for others on the platforms in which I had was bound to end. It was necessary, so I could walk hand and hand with destiny and purpose. I resolved to protect the new passion. Unlike dance, this passion joined a union with purpose; therefore, I will do what is in my power to prevent another loss. Like my clients, I, too, experience emotional and psychological benefits when I am relishing in my creative space. Not only am I transforming the physical with makeup and skincare, but I am also transforming lives by extending the feelings of positivity, strength, and a yes-you-can-do-it attitude. They pour into me while I am pouring into them. You will be amazed by who and what will grace life's path. Because I see and feel the transformation, I upped my game and creativity by embellishing every thought, which created my brand. In all things you do, seek more than passion, and have a sense of purpose. The pleasures from purpose will last a lot longer and help you understand and serve others while adding value to their lives.

Rashad's Identified Trauma, Challenges, and Barriers
Hopelessness, Loss, Not Good Enough, Relationship Trauma

Rashad's Journey to Wellness Story
Understanding my values and realizing my worth facilitated the birth of purpose. But it was not until I reached a pivotal moment in my life that the glimpse of purpose made its debut. And, no, it was far from delectable. But, you see, the journey of purpose discovery is neither a zap nor does purpose come easy. Sometimes you must go through some heartache in order to gain the self-awareness and knowledge necessary to activate a sense of purpose within you. In my own case, it was a 5-year abusive relationship. It was not just physical abuse, but also mental.

I had chosen someone with whom I thought I would spend the rest of my life. Up to this time, I had not experienced anything I could call traumatic except the death of my sister, who passed away at 18 during childbirth. I remember going from my sister's funeral straight to my graduation. It was tough. But I had such a tight loving family that I could weather the tragedy of that loss— through the love and support from my parents and siblings. However, when it came to this toxic, abusive relationship, it was much different—again, much more different.

Well, I had the option of remaining in my wreck or turning the pieces into valuable use for the better. Thank God I chose the latter. Had I not taken ownership of what I had gone through and worked through the trauma, no relationship of mine, whether personal or business, would probably have the capabilities to flourish. That experience birthed the purpose deep within me. It had been there all the while without me even noticing it, usually expressing itself in things I did so naturally, effortlessly, and with much relish.

Rashad's Old Way of Thinking—Negative Thoughts

I am not enough! This was the thought that often plagued my mind—"not enough for someone to love me again," blah, blah, blah. Although I have done the work to repair myself, I sometimes find myself questioning my qualifications, relevance, and competence. Still, I question if I am bringing enough to the industry. However, I have learned to speak the opposite of those negative thoughts whenever they creep in and make peace with not being everything or enough, for no one is indeed enough or all-sufficient. At best, we all are still striving towards perfection and pushing for higher grounds. In those moments of feeling "deficient," if we welcome the challenges with the belief in subsequent mastery, we are able to stretch and expand to new levels.

Rashad's Old Reactions and Behaviors

One of the things that quickly takes me back to old feelings is yelling. Anywhere at all, whether or not it is directed towards me, yelling makes me fretful and vulnerable. It triggers an internal shutdown, causing me to retreat into my shell.

Rashad's New Way of Thinking

Expansion and Confidence. First, I accept who I am: I am valuable and good enough. And I am poised to expand my capacity. While I know I have not arrived yet, I neither let that keep me bound to inaction nor do I beat myself up for the long way I still have to go. I keep moving and improving.

Rashad's New Responses and Behaviors

I have a daily affirmation that I say and share with other people regularly. It is precise and covers everything I believe. That is the way I maintain a new way of thinking.

The affirmative thoughts of more than enough develop behaviors and expand roads traveled. It motivates me to make small steps towards the things that I desire. It also keeps me in check when I seem to be drifting away from what I desire to manifest into my life.

Rashad's Restoration Tip

Life events have certainly shown, taught, and allowed me to thrive beyond my wildest dreams. I have picked myself up from rock bottom, starting life entirely over—away from my entire family—and building a more durable sanctuary. Through it all, I know for certain that success is achievable. You never know your strength until it is activated, usually through unsavory circumstances.

Rashad's Definition of Success

Success is contentment, peace, and happiness. That includes financial stability (being able to afford the things I need in life), relationships and friendship, and seeing healthy connections. Most importantly, success means that I am truly happy with the person I see each day I step out of bed, the person I see when I stand before my full-length mirror. Success is when I say to myself, "I am proud of you."

Rashad's Journey to Wellness Takeaway

The takeaway is to always find the lessons in every situation. Find yourself, honor yourself, and, most importantly, refuse to be responsible for the way people treat you. Still, you are most certainly responsible for your journey on the road to recovery, irrespective of the residue after the mistreatment.

Rashad Advises

In life, everything and everyone present signs. Do not allow clouded judgments to deny your worth. Uphold your values. No matter what, if something dishonors you in any way, shape, or form, address it. Have enough self-awareness, have an honest conversation, and choose what ultimately honors you first.

Journey to Wellness Practical Tool

Cognitive – Old Way of Thinking - Negative Thoughts
Instructions: Pause and take three deep breaths to clear the mind, then complete the exercise. List three negative self-thoughts you experienced during this chapter.

_____

_____

_____

_____

Emotional – Accepting Feelings and Emotions – Negative or Positive
Instructions: Pause and take three minutes to notice and connect with your feelings, then complete the exercise. Identify, list, and recite three emotions you are feeling at a particular moment. Be compassionate with yourself.

_____

_____

_____

_____

Cognitive, Emotional, and Behavioral – New Way of Thinking, Responses, and Behaviors
Instructions: Reflect on the questions throughout the chapter, explore new thoughts and desired changes. Rewrite the three negative thoughts listed above into positive thoughts.

_____

_____

_____

_____

Recite each rewritten positive thought three different times throughout the day. Remember to use a compassionate tone. Journal the times below.

_____

_____

_____

_____

Name three adjectives to describe how you felt after the positive self-talk exercise.

_____

_____

_____

_____

List three ways how you will think or respond differently to adverse challenges in the future.

_____

_____

_____

_____

PART THREE

Love Is

Proclaim:

Love is a beautiful mess.
It represents everything I WAS,
everything I AM, and everything I desire TO BE.
Each page turned tells a remarkable story that reopens the
heart.

I love "Love." I love its sound, its meaning, and its purpose. The mere thought of "Loving," being "Loved," or falling in "Love" feels so exciting and new. For me, expressing and sharing "Love" comes naturally. I do not think about it; it just flows freely. It feels like an abundant, limitless source. I feel the love in every little thing. In the embrace of a child, it is in the smile of a passerby, in the smallest of things, and the grandest of gestures. Love is everywhere. It consumes me fully and wholly. Giving the heart permission to love is like oxygen. It is a necessity. I cannot live without it. And it amplifies my energy vibrations to live life and find the strength in myself, to thrive in this ever so temperamental world. Like oxygen, Love is an element needed to create. Whether it is creating energy, memorable moments, or impeccable art, "Love" enables us to perform at our very best. And the best part of it all, love comes at no price. It may be hinged with conditions, but it comes to you every time you give it to others. In the wise words of Jenny from the block, "My Love Don't Cost a Thing."

Though dictionaries, scholars, musicians, poets, and even common men have tried giving various definitions and descriptions to "Love," no one will ever come close to capturing the entangled complexity of emotions stored in this Pandora's Box.

I misrepresented everything love is. In my past life, hearing the word "love" felt eerie. The slightest expression of love would send my mind running riot, and I would begin to suspiciously analyze things for trouble and other hidden meanings. Talk about cynicism. Do they really love me? Is this only for display? Are there any ulterior motives attached to this? Do I really love them? Although loving comes naturally to me now, that was not always my story. That is why I opened by saying I misrepresented love. Since my awakening, I look at certain people and quickly recognize in them the person I used to be. I see it in the way they talk and walk. By this, I can examine and reevaluate my life through a high definition lens, comparing or contrasting the old self with the new self, thereby improving by expunging any residual negativity and imbibing positivity.

The past has taught me the importance of being compassionate and patient with those who are learning the concept of love: the why and how, the do's and don'ts. What does it mean? Why do I choose Love? How do I Love, especially when it is not reciprocated? Here is the kind of attitude I have often confronted over the past five years.

Me:	*I love you.*
Them:	*I hear you. So, you love me?*
Me:	*Yes, I love you.*
Them:	*Are you sure?*
Me:	*Yes, I'm positive.*
Them:	*But I have doubts. It doesn't sound true; it doesn't add up.*
Me:	*What do you mean?*
Them:	*You, loving me. It can't be real, can it?*
Me:	*Oh, it's absolutely real.*
Them:	*Why me?*
Me:	*Why not you?*
Them:	*Out of all the choices in Atlanta, why me?*

Does the above dialogue sound familiar? (Now, not everybody reacts in those same words, but the above is a simple synthesis of their attitude.) What was your immediate thought when you read this exchange? What did you conclude from the conversation, a lack of worth? It is definitely nothing else but that—lack of self-worth. But I tell you what: feelings of unworthiness are not of sound mind. If you shall come across a similar conversation such as this, take heed, take time, and take a sedative because there is a long journey ahead if you choose to proceed.

One morning, my mother and I sat for breakfast after returning from the gym. She drank her morning coffee as I drank my post-workout shake. It is one of those wonderful moments and atmospheres in which I glean tremendous wisdom from her awesome cerebrum. As we talked, reflecting on special moments, with smiles and laughter, we talked about my recent endeavors. I mentioned that I had encountered individuals with stable jobs, great health, and even good money, but still, they were unfulfilled at the end of their day. Their sense of unfulfillment was almost intangible. Feelings of sadness, unworthiness, and guilt dominated their thoughts and characterized a general disposition that slowly but surely, plummeted their self-esteem. With low self-esteem comes a disregard for one's well-being. From our encounter, mom and I concluded that such people eventually fell out of love with themselves—or never fell in from the get-go. And what could be worse! **Know that Love Has Nothing to do with Feelings and Thoughts of Unworthiness.**

NOTIONS AND LIFESTYLE UNAGREEABLE WITH LOVE

None of the following is amenable regarding love (both love for yourself and love for others): feeling undeserving, overly critical, feeling not good enough, always regretful, constantly emotionally downcast, feeling of being a failure, constant fear, always forfeiting and compromising happiness, building insecurities, blaming others; the list goes on. Do any of these words describe you? Then let me tell you, this is not love. You are not in love with the self, or at least not as much as you thought. Do any of these words describe people around you? If yes, then let it serve as a wake-up call. It is important to recognize toxic patterns that drive love out of your life, but it is equally important to be wary of the toxicity around you. They can affect—or more correctly, *infect*—your chi, your soul's alignment, and your energy frequencies with their mindset in ways unknown. I am not saying to get rid of them, but you must devise a means of keeping your clothes unsoiled when walking on a dirt road.

Now that we know what Love is not let us explore what "Love" is. According to dictionaries, love is intense feelings of deep affection; it is profound, passionate, warm, and tender, coupled with personal attachments. But that is not all.

Dictionaries have up to 21 different meanings of this single word, depending on its use. The repeated keywords found in these definitions are passion and affection. I agree with them; however, I think love very much transcends feelings of passion and affection.

I represent everything love is. Though everybody may not accept my definition of love, for me, it is an experience I choose to carefully create. It is a choice. Every day, I willingly choose to fill my time with love. We are creations of love. If you are aware of this, you can actually create love, too. You are a creator of love because you are a creation from love. You can experience love everywhere and every time you blink; where it seems not to exist, create it. Because the source is within you, it can be replicated in others and your environment. Thus you experience yourself (love)—the creation and the creator. This is why, before I step out of the house or embark on a journey or even facilitate a meeting, the first step is to dedicate time, maybe an hour or so, to create an atmosphere of love. It is a preparatory stage where the soul and body are equipped to give and receive. I refer to this phase as "Getting Warmed Up." It is no different from any other warm-up exercise. Call it an icebreaker, if you may. The purpose of warming up is to increase flexibility and thus prevent injuries due to a strain or sprain. Like before getting into an intense workout, you warm up; love also requires warm-ups. Love warm-ups increase flexibility and reduce fear, nervousness, and anxiety while building trust and decreasing insecurities. Warming up slowly revs up the mind, heart, soul, and body to endure what is to come.

Understand that we respond differently to love because we generally perceive it differently. Some may catch the physical aspect of it and immediately find motivation in the sensorial signals, while some require cognitive stimulation in order to connect to it. And some even require both—physical and cognitive connections. Know that happens knowingly and unknowingly. Like the air, it is invisible all around us until you choose to activate it. Our conscious mind recognizes pronounced love. It accepts its own traditional expressions. Whether that is someone giving you a bouquet of roses with a simple "I love you" or treating yourself to a spa, the mind, one way or another, recognizes love and opens the heart to receive it. These experiences render a sense of security to you. These common gestures of love allow for healthy communication to develop where you and your partner discuss the needs that require fulfillment. Once the need is met, it boosts your self-esteem and consequently makes more room for self-acceptance. With that, you start to truly grow and accept the flaws, or theirs, in the relationship. This recognition and acceptance are another step in the right direction. The subconscious mind, meanwhile, experiences the unknown love, and it is vast. A simple rub on the hand makes your heart flutter, or a little "waiting for you every day" might have brought changes to your mood that you would not usually notice. These experiences offer indirect support, cause spontaneous humming songs and unconscious smiles or laughs, and ultimately create moments that the heart truly desires.

There are five "love languages": Words of Affirmation, Quality Time, Receiving Gifts, Acts of Service, and Physical Touch.

Whether your motivation is physical, emotional, or mental, intentionally choose to create love, first for yourself and then for others. Appreciate and say positive things to and about yourself. Here are examples of how you could use verbal expressions to nurture and reinforce inner positive image:

Look yourself in the mirror and say, "My, what a charming smile you have!"

Compliment yourself, "You look amazing today."
Say to yourself, "This new fragrance you're wearing is terrific. It smells pretty good."

Or even self-praise: *I am intelligent and successful. I am confident and inspiring.* And so on.

Tiny drops make an ocean. These refreshing showers sprinkled on tomorrow become fountains for you and for individuals around you in no time. Reassurances and reaffirmations such as these are like building blocks; you end up with an overflowing canal of love by the end of the transformative process to understand and explore everything love.

Creator + Choosing to Experience + Time = Creation

Love is everything I desire. If you have made it this far in life, your five or six senses must have been activated on some level, which means you are open to creating experiences if you choose. How is that so? It is so because someone or something at some point caught your *Attention.* Once your attention is given to a person, place, or thing, then you have chosen to create an experience. Now that the *creator* (you) *has detected the attention towards a thing*, it is a matter of deciding what to do next. Will you continue with this thought of attention or choose to move from that thought to action by investing time in this attention? If the decision is made to devote more time to create experiences with someone or something, the decision to devote now becomes the *Intention* of the act of giving attention to a person, place, or thing. As attention and time increase, care increases. Attention, time, and care create a favorable environment for love to breed. The choice to love by vicariously experiencing feelings, thoughts, and attitudes of another starts to manifest greater attention when it is nurtured. It offers emphatic support, which often increases the capacity to love. This might have been hard to digest but give it another read and truly absorb the words. They will help you understand how love is created and developed. Remember that attention and intentional care of the heart desires, with time, manifest greater love.

Increased Attention + Time + Care = More Love

Love is a widely researched and explored interest that many have attempted to understand since human creation. The dictionary may define love as an expression of passion and affection, but it is so much more. My love growth prompted me to develop an understanding of *Intention* and *Attention*. This elevated the tones of my emotions into unfamiliar terrains. I experienced a rollercoaster of a ride, sudden moves and shifts, uncertainty, and identity confusion. So for me, love was not always accompanied by passion; sometimes, it was met with forcible repositioning.

But like the air we breathe, we cannot escape love. We hear it, see it, feel it, witness it, and desire it. Love is you and me; it is simply our creation. We create unforgettable moments with whomever we please. Once love is given or received, it requires nurturing to maintain or grow. We offer our time and attention so that our love matures; when we offer more time, we give and receive greater attention.

Love is a Beautiful Mess - Introduction

Here is an interesting fact: The first time the Bible used the word "Love" was in an act of giving. Genesis 22:2 reads, "Then He said, 'Take now your son, your only son Isaac, whom you love, and go to the land of Moriah and offer him there as a burnt offering on one of the mountains of which I shall tell you.'" In this stated Bible citation, God had asked Abraham to give up his only son Isaac as an offering. The situation was as oxymoronic as a *"beautiful mess."* But there is a way around it. Another Bible verse is, "God so loved the world that He gave his only begotten Son." In these references, you can identify both passion and affection. Abraham had affection for his son, but it did not exceed the affection he had for God, and so he was ready to sacrifice his son to value the love he had for his Creator. So love occurs in versions and degrees, and the determiner is the *priority*.

I began working at the age of fourteen. Honestly, I cannot recall why I started so young, but thinking back, I felt I had a responsibility for my siblings. I cared for and loved them so much that I desired to provide for them. Their needs became before mine. That was the earliest form of sacrificial love I recall demonstrating. I am still not sure where, how, or when I began to love, but one thing is certain: I did not start self-love until recently. If I had to rank my loves several years ago, it would fall in this order: family, intimate relationships, God, me, and lastly, other material things. Do not shake your head; I know, I know I am a work in progress. I was just as surprised as you at these results. The ranking scale is based on my relationship with each one. I encourage you to assess and rank your relationships as well. You, too, would be surprised with your results if you are honest.

As I grew more in love with myself, it changed my ranking scale. Now it is God, the God in me (soul and spirit), my family, intimate relationships, and then other material things. Think about who or what gets most of your attention. This will help you in establishing a priority list. With your priorities in place, you can work towards reaching your divine purpose.

Love is a Beautiful Mess – Protection

Love is not always hearts, roses, birds, candies, swans, and doves. It is also struggles, yearning, sorrow, metamorphosis, peace, and the ability to say no. Did your parents ever say to you, "I beat you because I love you," or "This is going to hurt me more than it'll hurt you"? My mother was the disciplinarian in our house, and so my father never gave me a *"whooping"* (as kids call it) like most children. We were taught to accept it as a learning curve because it was simply better for us, in my mom's words. As a seven-year-old child, every time I got whipped, I was expected to look at my mother and think, "Because she loves me." When I just thought, *she just lost her raggedy mind?* my mind would quickly reset to default because I knew *she indeed loved me.* My mom assigned all my siblings and me certain household chores. Being kids, we were quite slothful about completing those tasks. Little did we know that because of this lack of urgency, she would explode. Since I was the oldest, automatically, I was deemed responsible for all the wrongs, so I bore the brunt of the havoc that ensued. My mom got hold of my dad's leather belt and whipped me to teach me a lesson. As I lay on my bed afterward, I thought to myself, with a sore butt and disoriented emotions, *how can this possibly hurt her more than it hurts me? She doesn't have an aching body; I do. If only I could swap bodies with her, I could easily bear her 'hurt'!* Here again, love is a beautiful mess. As a child, I did not enjoy the profound affection delivered via whippings. But now, as a mature adult, I understand that her deep affection, delivered through this form of discipline, was her love of protection. I also think about what could have happened if she did not show her love and affection in this manner. Disaster, sure bet!

Love is a Beautiful Mess – Attraction

Giving and receiving love is beautiful until someone expresses it uncannily. News flash! Love is not only associated with good emotions; it actually encompasses the good, the bad, and the ugly. For instance, ever heard the statement *Truth is bitter?* (Someone even made it rough by saying *Truth is a painful *itch!*) This happens when you are lost in a euphoric bubble and then comes reality (truth) and pokes it. Surely you were not prepared for this truth. But it takes love for someone to share it with you—and vice versa. Because our life stories differ, we become polarized; this polarity in close range can cause pain, disappointment, heartache, stress, and heartbreak. If you choose to love, you also choose to hurt. You cannot have one without the other. You can, however, enjoy one more than the other. Once more, we see the oxymoron—the beautiful mess—the paradox of love.

And how do we attract in the first place?

Do you believe in the law of attraction? I do. The law of attraction is the principle that whatever frequency you send out in the world using your thoughts, words, and actions are exactly what you get in return in life. You receive what you broadcast. If you are constantly thinking of worries, troubles, and toxic things, then that is what will be attracted. If you fill your life with happiness, joy, healthy friendships, and food, then the world and works of nature will give you more of that. Based on this law, we can conclude in simple terms: love answers our individual thought life. Thus, we attract our inner self even though the attraction may initially seem contradictory.

Remember the equations below.

Creator + Choosing to Experience + Time = Creation

Increased Attention + Time + Care = More Love

I hope you are following and connecting the dots. There comes a moment when two souls are aligned to engage physically. Though we exist in our own spheres, in separate vehicles, our minds work to send signals to the universe. For example, say you meet someone; before you know it, you all eyes connect, and metaphysical engagements take off into the atmosphere. Soul communication permeates expeditiously through the air like a flashlight, and before you know it, an unexpected turn of events comes after. It is so intense that it feels like running a 10K on Independence Day at the Peachtree Road Race. The connection passionately magnifies, generating unexpected emotions. The communication between twin flames rapidly charges the air gases, causing combustion that is bound to become a furnace. Fortuitous, you may say. But do you terminate? Heck no. The metaphysical dialogue continues. Things are going well now, and you may burst into flames at any moment. Words flow effortlessly. Big smiles continue body language, all gentle crest to more intense, beautiful levels. You listen and hang onto each other's every word.

Both of you walk down an open landfill during the fall, making imprints in brilliant green ryegrass. Beside you is the riverbank where the water current is in sync with the pace—or so you thought. You all are not alone; the birds and the bees, the clouds against a background of clear blue sky, as well as the wildflowers and dragonflies surround us. The river flows so tenderly, and on its clear surface, both images are mirrored, meshed together in captivating harmony. Sunlight penetrates through the towering trees. An abundance of wildflowers adds beauty to the scenery, not only for our enjoyment but also for the birds, the bees, and the dragonflies to enjoy and frolic.

Initially, 15 minutes were allocated for this experience, but you chose to increase the time to 38 minutes along the line, which caused *greater attention*, leading to greater love. The "take-home pay" of this adventure is that love can be unpredictable, unfamiliar, and governed by the law of attraction. It moves swiftly, evokes hope, and afterward advances confidently.

Love is a Beautiful Mess – Continuum

Love's "Pursuit" took birth from different color spectrums, but mostly shades of gray. The shades signify family, friends, oneself, jobs, promotions, vehicles, accomplishments, marriages, intimate relationships, and casual ones. My love was never black or white. It has always been both objective and subjective, based on evidence or probable cause. Factors and circumstances contribute to experiences that determine where love falls on the gray color wheel. More than a spoken word, love is more than a dictionary-defined term, more than an action or adjective, and even more than an emotion. Love is the highest form of self-transformation—metamorphosis at its finest.

The "Great Love Roller Coaster" takes you on journeys through all four elements: travel in air, on land, through the fire, and underwater. Chaka Khan says, "Through the fire, to the limit, to the wall." Understand that the elements play a crucial role in our lives. Combined or separately, they produce organic and inorganic matter that sustains us. Continuum love is life's energetic vibration ebbing and flowing in the pursuit of unifying and elevating levels of awareness. The deeper the dive, the higher the emergence. Sometimes, it went beyond my own comprehension because I could not think bigger or see myself without the identified love interest. I did not think bigger, and bigger was not taught. And as they say, birds of a feather flock together, so those who surrounded me were too limited in their scope or chose not to share the knowledge. I learned the art of bigger through shades of gray, both loving and disliking, and smiling and crying. For three and a half years, I denied parts of me only to meet and greet my authentic self. It was mind-blowing.

Love is patient, kind, understanding, forgiving, healing, gentle, and powerful. It is so strong that 1 Corinthians 16:14 reads, "Do everything in love." The statement became my mantra in January 2016 when my soul endured an unfair, unprecedented, unpredicted attack. Love is a beautiful mess. I write because it is my story. I write to help others because I have gone through all four elements. It is real; it is hard; it is crippling when you are unaware and unequipped. The only reason I managed to live another day is that I developed a comprehensive approach to health and wellness: 4R Model: *Reconnect, Remember, Reflect,* and *Reboot.*

Love is a Beautiful Mess – Conclusion

When you were born, you entered the world as a perfect replica of unconditional love. Fragile, soft, gentle, and innocent, you hoped every time you smiled, cooed, giggled, or cried, someone would smile, giggle, and cry with you. Over time and quickly, however, you learned that human love is not unconditional but rather conditional, and for some, undeveloped. Although we are descendants of a Creator who loves unconditionally, we are conditioned to love others with levels of restrictions and limitations. Furthermore, adding to the problem, we tend to spend little time and effort developing self-love, which creates voids hoping something or someone can potentially fulfill.

I love *love*, though it is a beautiful mess. But let us work together, with the hope that it will become less messy than yesterday. If you need assistance doing so, visit www.*lovespursuitatl.net*, sign-up for our Wellness Coaching Services, and start anew.

Journey to Wellness Self-Discovery Reflection

Define "love." in your own words.

_____

_____

_____

_____

Reflect on two love experiences and write your ending.

_____

_____

_____

_____

What attracted you to these love experiences?

_____

_____

_____

_____

How did they shape you along the way?

_____

_____

_____

_____

Do you experience self-doubt, anxiety, or stress about exploring your love experiences? Explain why.

_____

_____

_____

_____

Do you think this could be rooting from past trauma or an unfair experience? Explain why.

_____

_____

_____

_____

What will you do differently in the next love venture?

_____

_____

_____

_____

Dear Black Man

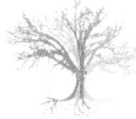

Proclaim:

*I pay homage to all Black Men
of influence in my life.*

Dear Black Man,

I pay homage to you! What are your fondest memories of the good times, Mr. Black Man? I ask about the good times because I do not recall any of the bad. Daddy, daddy, dad, father, pops, do you remember the good times? As a man and a father, some White Americans' attitude towards you is one of irreverence. They are deficient in veneration towards our shared heritage. Though you are not present to exercise your voice, I use mine to speak up— and speak your truth.

I regularly take a moment to doff my hat to you in the salutation of your strength and resilience in my prime. You have not only created my noble story but have salvaged it from being fictional and comprising imaginary tales and fables. The more populous race across the world attempts to generalize your story even though they stay aloof from your true history. In their amateur attempt at narrating your story, they make a caricature of your heroism; for it is indeed impossible for those who consider your melanin skin strange to understand the struggles and atrocities you endured. Instead of praising your strength, they are intimidated by it. Therefore, they exploited your fathers and grandfathers by employing them without pay to till their lands, in prison and slavery, for their selfish economic gain. The same greenfield your ancestors harvested was where they were slaughtered. And even now, they continue to imprison us, not by shackles and chains but with metals of handcuffs, bullets, and jail cells. Today, they maintain their old agenda by fierce brutality, coercion, and unparalleled injustice, just as they did to you when they escorted you down the green mile. But I live today in their presence, not only as their nemesis but also as a worthy fruit of your sacrifices.

My Black Man, you remain the one of three who has inspired greatness in me, though we have never celebrated Father's Day together, never thrown a football to each other, or never hugged. I hope to become the heir of your dreams, to step into your shoes, and birth your unacknowledged potentials. Although the question nags me whether I will become a finer version of you—whether I will be better or bitter—I face the future with optimism.

Decisive, Direct, Dependable – Black Man

Dear Black Man,

Opa-Locka city resembles an enchanted Arabian night. On Ali Baba Avenue, one of our hangout spots, always put me in Aladdin or an Arabian Nights scene. Well, technically, it was more of your spot than mine. I just liked riding and hanging with you and the fellas, and secretly I knew it was only a matter of time when you pulled out your overstuffed wallet filled with cash and said, "Go get something from the corner store."

My siblings and I would hop into the pickup truck, and away we went, headed from 175th Street and 22nd Avenue to Ali Baba Avenue. "Hey Dad, look, the pool hall is open!" You pulled into the parking lot. We walked across the street and entered the hall. Your name is on everybody's lips like it is a hit song. You turned, looked at me, and I already knew what was about to happen. You handed me a few dollars, and I ran to the change machine to exchange the dollars for quarters. I bust a U-turn directly to the

84

jukebox. Which 45-inch record do I play first, Marvin Gaye or The Temptations? The Temptations it is. Ain't Too Proud to Beg starts while you are shooting the breeze with the fellas, drinking knotty head (Seagram's Gin), and smoking Kool-Filthy King cigarettes. You looked over, and we were playing Atari's Centipede, Pac-Man, Galaxy, and Donkey Kong.

    Leaving the pool hall, we headed to Duval Street—"The Tree," as they called it—another one of our favorite hangout spots. "Dad, I know Kojak will be there." We pulled up, and sure enough, he is smoking cigarettes and drinking alcohol with a group of guys. They see us getting out of the truck and started with the jokes. They shout, "Hey Man, I see you stuck with the kids today." You laughed and responded, "Yeah, I have got my chillans." Dad, you know you were as country as hell, right? My siblings and I ran into the corner store to buy more potato chips and candy. We played tag around The Tree while you all were conversing and laughing as Kojak showed off his new Lincoln Town Car. That was just one of the many times I enjoyed bonding with my Black Man.

    I cannot forget when I landed my first job. I felt rapturous to be employed, to earn $3.35 an hour, scrubbing toilets and baseboards. You exuded pride for my sake. "My boy," you said. I do not know who was happier, you or me. But I was in a dilemma of transportation. My weekly work schedule consisted of Saturdays and Sundays from 6 a.m. to 2 p.m. Getting home was not an issue but getting to my workplace was since the Metro bus did not run early enough for me to arrive on time. I did not know how to ask for your help. "Dad, can you take me to work in the mornings?" "Sure, son!" you replied. It was that easy! You were a man of your words. Every Saturday and Sunday, you arrived on time to take me to work, except the one Saturday you overslept. The horn blew at 5:15 a.m., with me running out the door and greeting you with sleepy eyes. Although our conversations were not substantial, your presence and morale were sufficient for me to achieve my goals. Besides, I was not an early riser, so meaningful conversation at 5:15 a.m. was out of the question. That was apparent, for when you looked over to your right, you saw me sleeping with my head slightly pressed against the window. Dad, I could have thanked you for your love and support when

I had the time. However, fate was not cruel to me because the roles would soon reverse. You managed to work a full-time and part-time job and, yet, made sure I arrived timely at work every weekend. If this is not a representative of a direct, dependable, and decisive Black Man, then no human is such.

I picture you in my mind looking down from the clouds and cracking up over these stories. But I am not finished; there is one more. I hope you recollect this, dad. Every summer, you, mom, and my siblings distributed telephone books in our community. We drove to the warehouse, stacked the telephone books on the back of the pickup truck, and delivered Southern Bell Yellow and White pages door-to-door. Do you remember their slogan, "Let Your Fingers Do the Walking"? Both books were wrapped in a thick, plastic protective sleeve to safeguard them from outside elements. They weighed at least six to ten pounds. There we were, carrying them from porch to porch like the Incredible Hulk and Wonder Boy Robin. Though I was lean—and some may even say skinny—you could not tell me anything when I modeled your delivery skills. We relished this annual summer activity for many reasons. First, it created special moments—priceless. Second, it taught us the importance of working as a unit: we were our brothers 'keepers. Third, we learned the dignity of labor. Hard work pays off. Fourth, compensation felt good after completing a project. On top of that, we learned that money does not grow on trees, and we earned every dime.

Though America may attempt to qualify Black Men as "less than," Dad, I am here to protect and tell your story as my Black Man. You were not inferior to the military troops and veterans but were equal. While they were protecting our borders and supporting foreign nations, you were forced to fight domestic, racial wars, and social inequality to better our family and communities. Thank you for being direct, decisive, and dependable. Rest well. We will see each other one day, just no time soon.

Uncle – Black Man

Dear Black Man,

Dare a spirit lie that I forgot about you? No, never. For the life of me, I could never forget you. I also pay homage as I do to my dad, for you are a major weave in my story's fabric. Out of all the men in my life, I spent the most time with you, laughing and watching music videos. You remember that time we debated who the best artist of all time, Michael Jackson or Boy George and Culture Club, you remember? We stayed up all night going back and forth, and you sure won that debate. I am sorry to be the bearer of bad news, but just in case you have not heard, he is no longer with us. Or maybe you know better, for he is probably up there with you and dad sharing the same space. If so, I am sure all three of you are dancing around and moon-walking in the blue sky and on the puffy white clouds.

I cannot forget that time when I begged to watch The Best Little Whorehouse in Texas *with Dolly Parton, and you would not let me because you wanted to watch Michael Jackson on the Grammy Awards show. Do you remember that, my dear uncle? I ran and told Grandma, and she made you change the channel. OMG, you were so mad, but I will pick another time to describe the look you gave me that night. What could my little peanut-sized brain have known? But you knew Grandma did not play about her grandchildren. It is much like predicting who would win the 1996 Mike Tyson versus Evander Holyfield fight for the World Boxing Association heavyweight championship at the MGM Grand Garden Arena. Holyfield won by a TKO in round 11. I, however, won in round one within the first three minutes! BAM, I beat someone to the punch. I trust you are not still mad.*

By the way, thank you for helping me with my homework. Black Man, your intellect still amazes me. And I know you would be proud that I finished high school and graduated from college with three degrees and four certificates and started a business. It is easy to see our generational bloodline flows very well in me, with the same entrepreneurial spirit, determination, independent thinking, and card games skills (especially spades), but drinking spirits skipped my gene pool entirely.

I get sad at times when revisiting thoughts of you. Now that you are physically no more, I miss you terribly as I reminisce and tell stories of you as it seems to spell your name and walking past the places we visited revives the old scenes of you and me. Like I said to Dad, I am sure I will see you again someday, just no time soon. I still have your legacy to show the world and communities with other little Black boys to inspire.

With so much happening in the world, all calculated to thwart history, I use my voice to speak my Black Man's truth. We are living in a time with so much racial, social, and economic divide. We are so misrepresented. The words they use to describe us show their dismay and disconnect. The pictures painted are deceptive strokes heavily soiled in stereotypical disparity, perpetuating broken systems and causing institutionalized discrimination. The trickle-down effect is trickling too damn slow. The belief is that as the income rises at the top, it will lead to more jobs and less poverty for those at the bottom. America, check the facts because poverty still sits at our front doors. To be honest, many of us are displaced and do not "own" or have a front door. So, I speak to tell my Black Man's truths and experiences. For if I do not, then my story becomes cursed to be misconstrued.

I encourage those who know to do the same. Now, more than ever is an opportunity to pay homage to your Black Man—the Black Man who encouraged you; the Black Man who inspired you; he who changed your tire, paid your rent, bought your first pair of shoes, or provided you with various entertainment through his writing, acting, singing, rapping and athletic skills; the Black Man who pushed you beyond your circumstances to actualize a better future. He may not be a Malcolm X or a Martin Luther King, Jr., but along with these men, he also, within his own capacity, paved the way for you and many others. Theirs may be baby steps or giant steps, but we acknowledge every mile they walked in order to ensure that you and I are not hunted and lynched in our backyards as a sport for the world to see on video. They walked, marched, endured, and broke their backs to give us the life we are now living.

It is not just for them that they evoked actions, but for posterity, which includes us today. Your heroic deeds are the building blocks upon which the next generation will build to make a better version of you. Let your decisions be informed of its collective consequences, for the destiny of your generation hangs on them. They depend on you. Today you may well look back and discover the Black Men that empowered you, the Black Male ancestor that paved your way. To them pay homage. From them, draw inspiration.

As a child, I watched my father and uncle work tirelessly to provide for their families. Through thick and thin, anxiety within and acrimony without, they bestowed on me the virtues of hard work and kindness. They loved me enough to avoid imposing their opinions of mature personhood upon me but rather allowed me to develop into mine. I imagined my father's face at my Man of Tomorrow banquet and high school graduation. It is commonly reported that he was a man of few words, but his presence spoke volumes, and the entire block went silent at the rise of his voice. His voice made him seem like a one-man orchestra. He is a Black Man who needs no introduction.

Dear Dad,

Like a knight in a special military force, you answered swiftly each time I needed you. Knowing that a son needs a father to become a man, you exemplified a balanced mixture of confidence like dark roasted, blended coffee from **Urban Grind** *and* **Good Karma**. *You just cannot have one cup. Better yet, make it one cup with a double shot of espresso. You taught me to* *question my doubts and doubt my fears. Thus you built in me an adventurous spirit, vigor, and calculated risk. The weight of nine children neither broke you nor did your skin color shame you. When it seemed that your future inspired no hope, you started drawing hope from my future. Thus, just before the burden became too heavy, we were able to exchange roles successfully, and I became your Black Man and did what I could to relieve the pain and frustration. This is how our love weathered every storm 'til death called.*

I am yet to experience fatherhood for myself, but I have vowed to represent the freedom, love, laughter, and growth you bestowed unto me when it happens. A remarkable impression of security you engraved on the heart of mine and my siblings. 'Still now, though you are long gone, I still hear your voice behind me, and your laughter rings in my head. You are my alter ego; my ears remain sensitive to your spiritual vibrations, counsel, and guidance.

Dear Reader,

You have come too far, faced many obstacles, and experienced far too many disappointments on your journey to give up. No matter how things play out each day, reflect on the Black Man or Black Men in your life and draw strength from them. Continue to hang in there, for your work is not done. Payday is on its way. Now is the time to examine your heart and explore love, grief, and inspiration to understand the impact and influence your Black Man had or still has in your life. Find pictures or written words of him as a reminder of his contributions. It can be a family member, friend, neighbor, or celebrity. Pull from their strengths, learn from their weaknesses, and take full advantage of opportunities that can transform your life.

Our world right now is divided like never before. Our diversity and differences should unite us, not separate us. Be the reason why we come together, accept, and recognize our differences and turn them into our strengths. But due to the clever ploy of a few, these differences amongst us are exploited. Do not stand on the sidelines and just let things happen; instead, make things happen. Learn and unlearn. Once you start experiencing and learning things for yourself, you will discover all the lies and stereotypes you were fed up with until this moment. Actively participate in the campaign against social and economic injustices. This will feel like a reincarnation. You will feel enlightened. It will pave a path for a better future, and your children's future will spread like ripples to those around you.

My Black Man

Worthless coal
Earthy coal
Brittle coal
Dark coal
Black coal
Oh, hated coal!

But wait… Just like the coal…
Like the coal, Black, they throw you in the fire to suffer
Now in the fire, Black, you become all that they desire
For the stronger your heart
The greater your strength

They say, Black, you are of limited value
But why, Black, do they persecute you?

They curse you "dark" and unwanted
Yet in their fire, you shine red
Then they use your heat for warmth
Or they use it for cooking
And for smith, and your black for painting
Until, by slavery, you're brought to ashes
And they lie to your coming generation
That you did not know civilization
Because if your children knew the truth
They'd learn from you and become genius

The slavery is merely envy

The injustice is simply jealousy
Because they wish to have your melanin power
Which they lack, and thus are lower

But your child buys their lies
And as you die, so he too dies

You rose early, worked many jobs for small cents
And each night, it's near midnight before you sleep
Your shoulders hurt, and your back breaks
The kids see your smiles but not your aches
They grow up with love and strong like you
While they usher their gratitude with "Thank you."
They care for you until they lower you six feet down
They live bereft, filled with void and grief
And because they know not your story,
Someone else distorts their own history.
Thus, the legacy of the Black remains his slavery,
Until children of Black Men share their stories, just like me
I AM a Black Man birthed from a generational bloodline,
A bloodline of Rick Black History.

Journey to Wellness Practical Tool
Instructions: Pay homage to your Black Man by reflecting and journaling

Journey to Wellness Practical Tool

Cognitive – Old Way of Thinking - Negative Thoughts
Instructions: Pause and take three deep breaths to clear the mind, then complete the exercise. List three negative self-thoughts you experienced during this chapter.

_____

_____

_____

_____

Emotional – Accepting Feelings and Emotions – Negative or Positive
Instructions: Pause and take three minutes to notice and connect with your feelings, then complete the exercise. Identify, list, and recite three emotions you are feeling at a particular moment. Be compassionate with yourself.

_____

_____

_____

_____

Cognitive, Emotional, and Behavioral – New Way of Thinking, Responses, and Behaviors
Instructions: Reflect on the questions throughout the chapter, explore new thoughts and desired changes. Rewrite the three negative thoughts listed above into positive thoughts.

_____

_____

_____

_____

Recite each rewritten positive thought three different times throughout the day. Remember to use a compassionate tone. Journal the times below.

_____

_____

_____

_____

Name three adjectives to describe how you felt after the positive self-talk exercise.

_____

_____

_____

_____

List three ways how you will think or respond differently to adverse challenges in the future.

_____

_____

_____

_____

PART FOUR

Purpose and Design

Proclaim:

*PURPOSE is an
assignment designed to
enhance your life and the
life of those around you.
Take every step, every
breath, and every
decision with purpose in
mind. This attracts the
very thing the heart
desires, and you begin to
live and fulfill your goals
with a clear direction.*

Pause for a moment, and for about 30 minutes, ask yourself this question: "What truly is my purpose on earth?" Often, people give me the side-eye when I say, "Thank the Lord for the good and the bad." Shouting for joy is natural and easy when you hit the lottery, but your whole disposition is a far cry from that when your soul (character) is brought through a furnace. In other words, maintaining a positive attitude when you are happy requires minimal effort. There was a time when I invited many and all kinds of people into my life. This meant that a lot of energy entered my "house," and many were reluctant to flee. Some of it was positive, consisting of love, happiness, acceptance, and gratitude, while some were the polar opposite and filled with gossip, hurt, disease, fear, and worries. Regardless of whether the energy was positive or negative, each of those encounters brought its weight to bear upon my purpose. A true test of character is when I was in despair and had to find the will and courage to carry on and remain consistent. And that is something I could only do when a set purpose was identified.

You see, when you have disconnected with purpose, dear friend, life flips like a light switch—almost suddenly, and the difference is like the contrast of light and darkness. It feels like dancing on cloud nine, then suddenly, both your favorite dancing shoes and jeans disappear into thin air. But whatever our experiences, whether good or bad, awesome or painful (such pain that was never imagined), it is necessary to fulfill life's purpose.

In my contemplation of purpose through pain, I developed a deep understanding of purpose mechanisms, that is, the relevance of the said purpose and its significance to lives. When I had just begun my purpose-driven journey, someone incidentally asked me what my purpose was. Loudly and proudly, I always answered, "My purpose is to lead people in the direction of the utmost good." My passion was unmistakable, having felt the scourge of bad leadership. To be more forthright, this response came from a place of hurt and trauma, as my superiors did not always respect my gifts, thoughts, and feelings when they did not align with their political or social agenda. So, I found myself trying to please the unpleasable. Have you ever encountered such people in your life? You are either doing too much or too little, moving too fast or too slow, overachieving or underachieving; they are always dissatisfied with your performance. Ugh... managing personalities can drain your energy, but it is maddening when those involved are prima donnas with a little or too much power. The excruciation is like daily penance!

In my experience, these are simply common signs of immense insecurities on the parts of those bosses. And people with such insecurities make themselves feel better about it by undermining their abilities. When you start feeling you are not enough for someone or someplace, it is a good indication that you have outstayed your welcome or were never welcomed in the first place. Take ownership of your destiny and therefore execute informed decisions. Determine to conduct yourself with healthy behaviors and a sound attitude, and close those chapters. Let me be clear about what I mean by "close the chapter": I am not suggesting to divorce or resign; I am simply saying that you should be clear and concise on exactly what you are feeling and experiencing. If you show ownership before describing what you own, it can drive you further into unknown territories. The more you are equipped to describe and understand your soul journey, the closer you move towards your purpose. Eventually, you will realize that purpose is not solely about you; it is an assignment designed to enhance the lives of those around you and maybe the world. It is then that your purpose becomes mine, yours, hers, his, its, theirs, and ours. Most of us desire the same things, such as happiness, family, love, and wealth; however, we all take different paths to reach our end goals.

Purpose is a universal human need. Without it, life is meaningless, and it will be challenging to find something as precious and necessary as happiness. The incoherence between what we are, what we desire to be, and what we do with life is one of the leading causes of personal dissatisfaction. Purpose provides the ultimate reason to thrive when the environment is at its best to pour directly into your reserve. The seed is sacred, the soil is cultivated, the water is purified, and the sun is vibrant, exuding Vitamin D. It is the right season to plant your seed and build good relationships. As my pastor would say, "This is good ground." The proper season will ensure that you have the time to commit and trust the process to find or continue your walk in purpose.

Purpose does not appear overnight. It does not come without yelling, tears, disbelief, and a cuss word or two. Also, it is not meant to be compared to someone else's destiny. Stay focused on your purpose, and let destiny assign others their special mission to fulfill. About six years ago, I wanted my doubts and anxieties to disappear with the flick of a magic wand in the hope that my fate would await me that year. Well, you know, that did not happen. I prayed and prayed and waited and waited. One of the most frustrating things in the world is to pray in and out of season and not receive the results of which you have prayed. When I learned that God is on His time and not mine, I sought other sources and fronts to serve as tangible inspirations and spaces to pursue life's purpose until He shows up. At the time, it was **Love's Pursuit**, family, community, hobbies, and volunteerism. Participating in purposeful activities can help reconnect you with the self and give life meaning. Once found and defined, purpose may appear immutable. But circumstances will arise that may lead to consider making substantial changes in its essence. That is, purpose is likely to vary over time and, undoubtedly, change at different stages of life. Therefore, purpose will not look the same as it did in your youth, the same in your relationship, or the same when you retire. In my experience, I learned that purpose is within; you just have to activate it.

Over the past few years, I have run into countless brick walls, glass doors, and turbulences. Nevertheless, I have persisted. Specifically, last year, many chapters of my life almost reached their conclusions. To give you an idea of what took place before my reinvention, join me on the Cedar Point's Thrill Dragster traveling at 120 miles per hour, throwing you into a twist before racing to the finish line. But for me, there was never a finish line for months on end. I experienced one huge loss after another. I remember being emotionally numb at one point. This is when I birth the 4R Model: *Reconnect, Remember, Reflect,* and *Reboot.* The excavator began deep digging, moving, and transporting confusion and hurt to the sanitation landfill in those moments. The process was progressive, and each dig left huge gashes in what I had thought to be a solid foundation. It forced me to ask questions like, "Who am I? Why do I feel this way? How did I get here?"

But as I engaged more in self-talk, I started having a conversation with God. And thus, in the next months, I began to gain strength. Not long after, clarity and realizations entered my mind. There was a realization of purpose in my life, and I met it with profuse joy. Purpose was, and continues to be, the central motivator of my life. It is the reason that I usually wake up every morning to live another day. When you realize that purpose is an assignment bigger than yourself, you begin to operate with an inclusion mindset, make innovative decisions, rise above unanticipated challenges, and gain a sense of direction. I have bid adieu to doubt and uncertainty—these did reach their conclusions. And what a miracle! "I WALK with purpose, and in fact, I AM purpose."

Try new things. Go on adventures. Meet exciting and inspiring people. And, if there are none around, meet me!

Hi, my name is D.B. Marshall. It is a pleasure to make acquaintance with you.

Joint inspirational souls will only inspire big, bigger, and the biggest dreams imaginable. I encourage you to parse out your priorities. Prioritizing will give a clear indication of what you desire in life. It also reduces stress and increases productivity, supports relaxation, and motivates.

Joining support groups that share similar struggles will afford you healthy companionship and even bring you the eureka moment you long for. A single breakthrough moment may be all one needs to get through hardships. *Be the Purpose!*

Journey to Wellness Self-Discovery Reflection

Define purpose.

_____
_____
_____
_____

What is your purpose? Describe in three or fewer sentences.

_____
_____
_____
_____

How are your priorities connected with your purpose?

_____
_____
_____
_____

Who or what do I value most in life?

_____
_____
_____
_____

What inspires me most?

_____
_____
_____
_____

Which celebrity, scientist, athlete, or innovator is my role model? Why?

_____

_____

_____

_____

What has hindered my path in the past? How do I manage or terminate it?

_____

_____

_____

_____

How do I replace my bad habits with better, more productive ones?

_____

_____

_____

_____

How do I make peace with those around me who demean me?

_____

_____

_____

_____

Define mindset. What is the difference between mindset, lifestyle, and purpose?

_____

_____

_____

_____

Journey to Wellness Practical Tool

Instructions: Use this blank canvas to explore your purpose. There are no right or wrong answers.

_____
_____
_____
_____
_____
_____
_____
_____
_____
_____
_____
_____
_____
_____
_____
_____
_____
_____
_____
_____
_____
_____
_____
_____
_____
_____
_____
_____
_____
_____
_____

Pursuit of Purpose

The path of least resistance
Is more seductive than Delilah.
Who wants to go through strain and stress?
Pushing boulders uphill with bare shoulders,
And all the while coming across as maverick,
Your admirers now reckon you brain-sick
For charting a course unknown, "the road not taken"?
Having found your purpose, all along hidden.
And because your dream is unfamiliar,
Dissuaders make excuse that success is rare;
Besides, your journey's long, full of obstacles.
Stay with us, they urge, let us tango and tangle.
Heed their sweet talks, you lose focus, your dream dwindles.
But if you jilt all enticements
And predicted predicaments
And persevere through the road of hard rocks,
Eyes fixed on the crown, enduring your cross,
Then yours is the glory after the story,
Where former seductions are but vanity.

If you are surrounded by people who genuinely care, I am confident, at some point, they have suggested that you work toward finding a work-life balance. And, sometimes achieving this is not easy, especially if you are a person of color. The reality is that as a community, we are working three to four times as hard to find our happy place. Life for people of color in America has never been easy. Even when we are giving our best, some only highlight our worst. We are raising families, working multiple jobs, and paying off student loans while managing stressors, emotions, depression, hypertension, diabetes, cancers, kidney diseases, and more. Sometimes, I ask myself if being a person of color in America is bad for my health. Next, Edward Drake II briefly explores occupational wellness and his experience to achieve work-life balance and the American dream. You will read how Edward fought through the odds to improve occupational wellness by staying motivated, working towards a purpose, accomplishing goals, and loving the work to change young people's lives. Ladies and gentlemen, I introduce Edward Drake II.

Occupational Wellness

Meet Edward Drake II

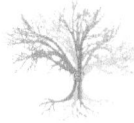

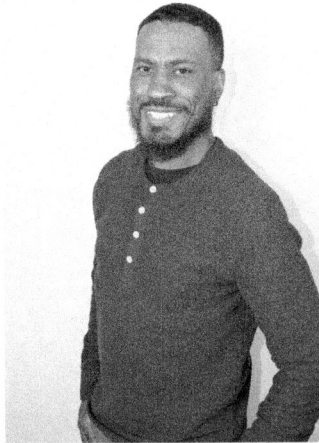

Proclaim:

*Never Stop Dreaming,
Believing, Persevering, and Giving Back.
Though I lost my dream, I found my purpose.*

Introduction

I hail from Ohio. Raised in a single-parent home with one brother and two sisters, I grew up versed in sports and even had the opportunity to pursue both football and track on a collegiate level. In addition, I have always had a passion for business and entrepreneurship. I am a creative soul who creates in the face of risk and uncertainty, for my purpose is to help others through profit growth and opportunities. Purpose guided me to become the founder and CEO of the YNOTT? (Youth Needing Organ & Tissue Transplants) Foundation and reside as the President at YNOTT? ME Enterprises, which is a consulting and investment firm. Why not me? Why not you? Besides the rewarding profile above, I am also a kidney transplant recipient. I must say that I have beaten many odds in life and will simply keep at it and inspire others to give their very best shots no matter the circumstance.

Edward's Identified Trauma, Challenges, and Barriers
Denial/ Rejection, Single Parent Household

Edward's Journey to Wellness Story

I was diagnosed with End-Stage Renal Disease in the summer of 2016. It was during my sophomore year at college as I was pursuing a life-long dream of playing football. During one of those routine physical examinations, the doctors were so shocked by my blood pressure level (reading 248/119) that I was immediately rushed to the emergency room. And on that day, my life changed forever. At the height of my athletic and academic careers, I literally went from a college campus straight to a hospital bed in the prime of my life with kidney failure.

During my dialysis treatments, I often griped and complained to myself, questioning, "Why me? Why now?" Later, a retort started springing in me, "Why not you?" Then it transformed into inspiration: "Why not apply your survival experience into an offer of hope to others who are in a similar circumstance of organ failure and other life-threatening illnesses? Why not teach them how to fight as you are doing?" Such a challenge emerged on my inside in spite of my pains! And through pain, fear, and faith, along with a passion for helping youth like me, I was inspired to form the YNOTT? Foundation. Success was given a new meaning.

Once the Lord revealed His purpose for my life through what I was going through and blessed me with a platform (YNOTT?) to help others in similar pain, fear, and confusion of such diagnosis, my attitude towards my situation changed—and so did my *altitude* in life. I was elevated above the "me only" to the "you as well" order of life. I then stopped complaining and started striving to bless others. I never knew that I, too, would receive healing from the same support groups I was hosting for pediatric transplant patients and their families. The feeling of touching lives along this journey has been priceless. These people include my family and friends, The YNOTT? Foundation, the various groups I volunteered with (namely, Lifeline of Ohio, National Kidney Foundation of Ohio, Nationwide Children's Hospital, etc.), and a lot more.

Edward's Definition of Success
Success means fulfilling your calling and encouraging others to do so as well. This is what ultimately guarantees happiness and peace in life—which should be a must for everyone because life is short.

Edward's Restoration Tip
Being happy and fulfilled.

Edward's Journey to Wellness Takeaway

Never give up! God has a purpose in your life. Seek and be obedient to what God calls you to do and pursue. You cannot have a testimony without a test.

Edward Advises

Proverbs 3:5-6 (King James Version): "Trust in the Lord with all thine heart; and lean not unto thine own understanding. In all thy ways acknowledge Him, and He shall direct thy paths."

Journey to Wellness Practical Tool

Cognitive – Old Way of Thinking - Negative Thoughts
Instructions: Pause and take three deep breaths to clear the mind, then complete the exercise. List three negative self-thoughts you experienced during this chapter.

_____

_____

_____

_____

Emotional – Accepting Feelings and Emotions – Negative or Positive
Instructions: Pause and take three minutes to notice and connect with your feelings, then complete the exercise. Identify, list, and recite three emotions you are feeling at a particular moment. Be compassionate with yourself.

_____

_____

_____

_____

Cognitive, Emotional, and Behavioral – New Way of Thinking, Responses, and Behaviors
Instructions: Reflect on the questions throughout the chapter, explore new thoughts and desired changes. Rewrite the three negative thoughts listed above into positive thoughts.

_____

_____

_____

_____

Recite each rewritten positive thought three different times throughout the day. Remember to use a compassionate tone. Journal the times below.

_____

_____

_____

_____

Name three adjectives to describe how you felt after the positive self-talk exercise.

_____

_____

_____

_____

List three ways how you will think or respond differently to adverse challenges in the future.

_____

_____

_____

_____

PART FIVE

Focus on Your Focus

Proclaim:

*Focus on Character Development,
Commitment, and Leadership.
Power up and Approach the Day
with Great Zeal!*

In nostalgia, I have amazing memories of how my personality has fared amidst challenges over the years. Though much was expected of me, life as a child was exploratory, fun, memorable, and carefree. Being the eldest of four, the crap-load of responsibilities was overwhelming. I did not know it then, probably because I did not perceive my duties as "work." (Thanks to my mother, who inculcated the dignity of labor into my psyche!) But from what my memory serves me, it was a lot. Mom always seemed to have had a SONny-do-list waiting for me. I was responsible for ensuring the house was clean, and everyone's homework was done. In addition to the sense of honor we derived from work, our labor sometimes came with its own pleasure. Apart from washing dishes, I also remember washing our clothes and hanging them on the clothesline when it was age-appropriate. That is right! We hung our clothes on a wireline in the backyard. This was usually the practice unless it rained. When it did, then plan B was implemented: the clothes were spread out on an indoor wooden drying rack. It was three tiers and provided roughly 27 feet of drying space. When we walked into the room, the detergent fragrance permeated throughout the house, smelling like fresh, clean, sweetness with lilac and cherry blossoms.

A dollop of gratitude is owed to my mother because she promoted self-discovery. Her attitude in my upbringing generally encouraged an acquiring insight to bloom into and cultivate my own character. Yes, there were a few times she challenged my idiosyncrasies as the concerned parent she was, but she mostly extended me enough rope knowing that rather than tending to preposterous obstinacy, I was just on the path of self-discovery and self-determination. Mature for my age, I approached most things with deep thought, consideration, passion, and compassion. I rarely fussed or fought the idea of who I was or what I desired to accomplish.

All the foregoing said I must confess to my limitations, too—my inhibitions. Growing up as a child, there were things that I never questioned because of the enjoyable safety and nurturing state of my immediate environment. But this is not an excuse. I totally own my flaw of succumbing too quickly to simplistic objections. Society did put a damper on my innocent curiosity, which should have been a portal into higher understanding and early discoveries. Yet, it was ultimately my undeveloped soul that caused my stuntedness.

Focus on Character

It is often said that if you want to change the world, begin by cleaning up and organizing your room. My character development journey was through diverse experiences that offered phases of dreams, lessons, and self-awareness. These occurred through family gatherings, pilgrimage, annual delivery of telephone books, and my genuine feelings and responses to issues or priorities, rather than being constructed by others'opinions on how I should feel or was supposed to feel. Whether or not one considers them consequential, these experiences of mine were the ingredients that imbued resilience, of which my success is a testimony.

This is not to say that I have already arrived. The truth is that the journey is ongoing. As Philippians 3:14 reads, I press toward the mark for the prize of the high calling… The more I develop, the more I create—and, in fact, the more I am myself recreated. There should be a continuity of developing the character that perfectly mirrors your beliefs and value systems. Awareness of one's beliefs and values holds one accountable and compels one into a life of indirect and direct characterization. To develop character, you must know where you have been, where you are going, and what you are willing to do or not do in order to get there. In other words, you must have a strong sense of self, value, and healthy boundaries.

Character building should not be a product of who others think you should be but who you desire to be. This is not to say you should be averse to advice or recalcitrant even when in error. Since no one is an embodiment of all knowledge and we are all prone to corrupt information, individuals must be open to learning new things, unlearning the untruths, and relearning crucial information. This calls for objectivity. This will enable change and expand a nobler character. Enrich your life with things learned and be intentional with the things that need shedding. Character change is possible when you pinpoint misconduct that holds you back, causes losses or incites harm. Just remember to practice positive thinking, and character development will build your unique three-dimensional character with depth, personality, and motivation.

Focus on Commitment

The word "commitment," like discipline, sounds like a lot of work. So at first glance of the above heading, some people become exhausted instantly or begin to experience anxiety. This is because not many people welcome perspiration—an imagery of work, which is to what commitment speaks. Think of having to couple two planks together and do it by hammering a nail through them. You must hit the nail, not once, but over and over and over again until almost perfect is achieved. That is commitment. Commitment does not come easy for some, and it can be scary and challenging, but it remains crucial. Commitment entails that one stays focused on one's pursuits. It is a conscious agreement between the mind, soul, and body. It compels one to dedicate the "self" to tackling matters with great zeal. Without commitment, the journey will not render lasting change. This is because nothing great happens overnight; one must consistently engage oneself in a specific endeavor to one's goals and one's priorities. Giving up midway or switching lanes before seeing things through will likely restart the process because a fundamental blunder would have been thereby committed and the entire success nullified. The thought of how far you have come in your struggle is capable of keeping you focused. Additionally, think about the joy of eventual fulfillment through continued commitment. It will inspire you every day.

When I learned of my chronic kidney disease diagnosis in 2012, I was confused. The bargaining stage of grief took full effect. Me? Is this really happening to me? No, it cannot be me! I am an avid runner, weightlifter, and athlete. I worked out four to six times a week and had never experienced hypertension, diabetes, or high cholesterol. Due to the diagnosis and shift in my health, kidney preservation added another stop to my journey. But this time, unknowingly, it was not a pit stop. The quick stop became a bypass that led to endless interstate connectors. Like "Atlanta Spaghetti Junction," it takes either a kind, supportive trucker who allows you to change lanes on the highway in front of them or a miracle to decrease the crowded, overlapping roads known for its constant bumper-to-bumper traffic. One never knows what will happen from one day to the next. To confront my fears and negative thinking, I gave myself three commitment options. I could commit to doing nothing, commit to kidney or renal failure, or commit to kidney preservation and reversal. I chose to commit to the latter, which is also my new normal: #iamakidneypatient. Focus on commitment, unwavering commitment, as it creates mutual trust between you and the desired outcome.

Focus on Leadership

When people think about leadership, oftentimes, the perception is high-ranking professionals with a pack of mentees or subordinates following after them. I challenge you to look at it from a different lens besides this stereotypic stance. Try leading yourself for a change. Set a path and build a passionate vision toward the creation of something that represents the new self and lead with conviction. Have a picture of the vision, imagine the person you aspire to become tomorrow and walk in that image!

The vision of an effective leader is always clear, organized, and directional. In other words, your goals must be defined. You cannot beat the air and fight without purpose; else, you will soon become frustrated. When you are clear about the destination, you will have direction and make a course correction if necessary. This way, you set a pace for others who come after you who may not know better and seek guidance.

Leadership is a magnificent quality to have, no matter in what spheres of life you exist. The ability to engage in a team and delegate to others firmly and deftly says a lot about one's character. It says that you can achieve an objective in a given timeframe, work cordially with others, know how to bring people together to accomplish tasks, and, therefore, welcome diversity and the idea of coexistence and harmony. Such quality does not go unnoticed by peers and superiors.

But even before your leadership prowess finds expression in the community or professional and business fields, it helps to identify personal issues and how to govern them. Your work will eventually speak for itself, and new opportunities will emerge or emanate. Therefore power up and lead your path to victory. When people turn their backs on you or fail to show up during struggles, they still forge ahead. Be your own motivator, inspiration, and coach. But when push comes to shove and you desperately need a cheer-LEADER, call me; I will cheer you on.

Three Ways to Gain or Regain Focus

Focus – Awaken with Mindfulness

Mindfulness is a cognitive process or state achieved by focusing on the present moment, the here and now. It is the ability to "be" without self-evaluation and moving from the past to the present for a second, a minute, or an hour. One common mindfulness practice is meditation. Mindfulness helps calm, acknowledge, and accept thoughts, feelings, and bodily sensations. The process happens without interpretation or judgment. The more it is practiced, the more one becomes aware. Practicing mindfulness includes, but is not limited to, sitting, walking, silence, paying attention, breathing methods, and self-acceptance. Mindfulness has the power to decrease internal threats and accusations. It helps to reveal and decipher between the hunter and the hunted. Before you know it, clarity emerges, and truths are affirmed. We are always in pursuit of reaching our goals, but how can we if we are running from ourselves. It is important to journey through uncomfortable places—**Love's Pursuit**—if happiness is your true desire.

As I previously stated, everything begins with a thought. Let me rephrase it, and hopefully, this message penetrates deeper. "Happiness begins with a thought." So many of us unconsciously are only living because we are on "life support." We are dragging around inconspicuous portable ventilators in an attempt to live an average life. But here is the bombshell: people on life support do not always recover. They may or may not regain functionality to breathe again. So as the cliché goes, "Give me my roses while I am living." I say to you, make time, meditate, and focus on breathing with the intent to align and awaken the self, so you can pull the plug—the life support plug, that is. The objective is to move from cognitive dependency to cognitive independence. It is time to breathe on your own, on your terms, and with great intention and attention.

Remember, pacing is key! Develop a plan to invest in yourself. It does not matter whether it is short- or long-term, whether it is big or small, attach it to focus until you are exactly where you are supposed to be. After each meditation exercise, it is helpful to first observe yourself in all shades of light: what you desire and what is blocking your energy source. In my case, I desire to focus more on the art of saying "no" and concentrate fully on adventures close to my heart that pour into my life as I pour into others. Therefore, I affirm: I free myself from soul-draining projects and focus on my soul-elevating enterprise.

Focus – Mental Focus

Mindfulness also helps with mental focus. Mental focus is a point where we direct our thoughts on a particular aspect of a circumstance or situation. It is the ability and skill to focus the intention on our attention. Together with physiology, it is one of the two main tools to help manage our moods.

How does it work?

Mental focus operates like a camera lens: if you focus on something in the foreground, it blurs everything into the background. Of what is obscured, you can no longer grasp the background details, and the focus becomes solely on you, like the portrait setting on a smartphone. What is out of focus loses its importance until it is no longer considered or even forgotten. Our brain has a similar device called the Reticular Activating System (RAS). RAS denotes that an aspect of the brainstem reticular formation executes a pivotal role in maintaining behavioral arousal, consciousness, and motivation. When the alarm is received and sounded, the conscious part of the brain recognizes the source and addresses the issue in question. RAS is useful because it speeds up our tasks to prioritize the attention needed to focus on our thoughts. RAS directs our attention to what arouses and interests us at that moment on the information most relevant and minimizing everything else. Therefore, keep in mind that our thoughts influence our moods.

Thoughts and moods.

Focus on your focus and pay close attention. When an individual unknowingly focuses on what is not working, life becomes a struggle, more complicated, scary, and cognitively dangerous. Mental focus can significantly affect our moods and emotions if there are no active tools to help us understand and heal. Use the tools in this book and focus on gaining practical experience. Humor me and try this exercise. Focus more on what your mind is absorbing from a favorite reality show or television series, such as the Housewives Franchise. It will divulge some unaware truths. Two of my favorite reality shows are *RuPaul's Drag Race* and *Marriage at First Sight*. I have yet walked away without receiving a positive message or being elevated. However, I cannot say this about much of reality television. Listen, I understand that sometimes entertainment allows us to escape, but do not get stuck in their fantasies or yours. Snap out of it! *Focus on Your Focus* and minimize and manage the overexposure of negativity highlighted on your media platforms.

Focus – The Power of Questions

In many situations, particularly these days, we are experiencing health emergencies and disparities due to coronavirus. It is prudent that we manage our thoughts and filter through negative information as much as possible. Some of those negative thoughts may consist of safety, helplessness, anger, sadness, and the inability to cope. While I completely understand these feelings and emotions, focusing on the negative creates a breeding ground for the negativity that can affect emotional balance and well-being.

How can we focus on useful thoughts? How do we redirect our attention to focus and shift more positively? Our minds are exceptional resources and are programmed to seek answers to the questions we ask ourselves; for this, it is essential to ask meaningful, relevant questions, which will result in useful answers. Limited questions will only produce limited solutions. Do you see yourself as limited? I do not think that you do. So ask relevant questions until you find the answer. There is always an answer. It may not be the answer you desire or the timeframe in which you wish to receive it, but there is always an answer. Sometimes the answer is no answer at all—dead silence. But can we accept silence as our answer? Speaking from personal experience, the answers surround us; we just have to raise our awareness vibration and look, listen, and feel the heavenly message being communicated. There are two categories of questions: the "why" and the "what/how."

"Why" questions

The "why" jumpstarts the understanding of the outcome. Questions like "Why me?" "Why did it happen?" and "Why can't I?" evoke myriad emotions and are useful in the beginning. It is comparable to brainstorming in that you list all the ideas or reasons in the order in which they occurred to you. It lays the foundation. However, this phase is short-term. We seek clarity to understand the intent or motive behind the action that left us bewildered and confused.

"What/How" questions

The *"what and how"* are more practical and functional than the "why." Questions such as: "How can I become a better person thanks to this?" "What would I gain from the present circumstance?" "How can I be useful in this situation?" "How can I have fun?" "How can I turn this negative experience into a learning lesson?" It is powerful to point out arrangements and actuate all your interior assets.

Journey to Wellness Self-Discovery Reflection

List three distractions in your life.

_____

_____

_____

_____

How can you change the distractions into purposeful connections?

_____

_____

_____

_____

List three positive, powerful characteristics that you possess.

_____

_____

_____

_____

List three characteristics you desire to develop.

_____

_____

_____

_____

What is the reason for the lack of your character development, if any?

_____

_____

_____

Do you accept your reality and work towards a better tomorrow or keep blaming things and circumstances for this lack thereof? Explain.

_____

_____

_____

_____

How do you move on from here? Write guided steps that will move the needle.

_____

_____

_____

_____

Possess Your Soul

I tell you one sure way to have your cake and eat it, too.
But first, you must quit running, chasing shadows, and admit,
Like you would before a witty judge, your guilt, in the court of conscience
For years of boot-licking, people-worship, pity-party, hiding in timid dress,
For each of those times, you sold yourself in exchange for nada,
Smearing contempt on yourself when rejected by a significant other,
Going low like a worm and hibernating for years in the mud and scum of
life—
For each of those times you wasted in regret—you are guilty of homicide.

As a water drop consumed in a hot frying pan,
So are you when you abandon your life for another's plan;
For when you are rejected, there is nothing left to do.
But as an ocean with multiple tributaries,
So are you when you own your choice and choose your destiny;
If rejected, you may not be aware; indeed, you had your cake and ate it too.

While interviewing Rashad Terry during this project, he made a powerful statement that will follow me to my grave. Rashad said, "You can't run from purpose. It follows you." Although I have not knowingly or intentionally run from problems, I am guilty of abandoning pivotal moments in my life for someone else's plan. When your actions or reactions are out of proportion with your circumstances, it is a strong indicator that you are out of alignment. You may ask, "How do I realign with my soul purpose?" One way is to commune with nature. Nature is known to have a calming effect. It is sure to guarantee and engage all of

126

your senses. Whether it is the sound of water, breeze of fresh air, or smell of the trees, nature has healing properties that can renew our souls. One of my future wellness goals is to perform a spiritual nature cleanse. I know you are like, "Huh?" For me, a spiritual nature cleanse is openly standing in the rain wearing swimming trunks, praying and chanting, allowing each drop to eradicate toxins, disease, and negativity symbolically. Jewlz's story ties nicely with this message. It illustrates internal conflicts, environmental disadvantages, and coping techniques that saved and developed her soul, which deepened her "selful" spiritual embodiment of love. Without further ado, I introduce Jewlz Shaw.

Soul Wellness

Meet Jewlz (SunGoddessBruj) Shaw

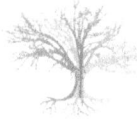

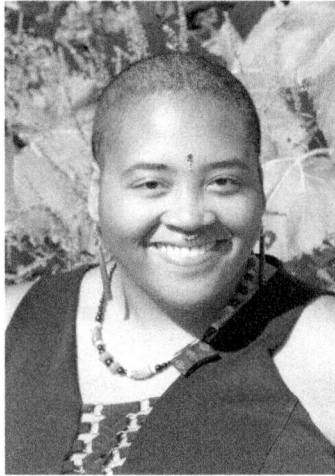

Proclaim:

*I am that I am and will always be exactly who I am meant to be:
I am daughter of Ra, devotee of Ma'at, and Warrior of Auset,
that 'selful' spiritual embodiment of LOVE!*

Introduction

Hi, my name is Jewlz. I was born and raised in Wisconsin, a state fueled by racism. Milwaukee, the city I lived in, is one of the most segregated cities in the country in terms of race and poverty. Even though I never grew up in "the hood," there was never a lack of fear. At the tender age of six, I was molested by one of my brother's friends. This situation led to being outcast by my entire family and group of friends, being my first experience of loss. I attended good schools, where I experienced racism from the White teachers, going as far as my third-grade teacher calling me a nigger! Despite these challenges, I was the emcee at my elementary Black history program, played an instrument, and was a cheerleader. These experiences provided me with a sense of hope that was taken away when my house burned down.

My dreams of becoming a nurse led me to attend a middle school in a very unsafe neighborhood. Due to the number of fights there, a situation occurred where two adults came up to the school to fight a student in which I ended up being physically assaulted as well. I was then transferred to a school in a safer neighborhood, but I was once again around racist teachers. I was almost expelled due to my teacher calling the police and falsely accusing me of threatening her. Due to the number of suspensions I racked up, I could not walk across the stage or even attend my eighth-grade graduation. So now that you know my backstory, let us continue through this journey together.

Jewlz's Identified Trauma, Challenges, and Barriers
Childhood Trauma, Loss, Anxiety and Depression, Unsafe, Racism, and Fear

Jewlz's Journey to Wellness Story

Wellness is all about balance, which to me is found in living a righteous life. A "righteous life" is not determined by what man or religion says is right or wrong, but instead according to your values and morals. Although I did not always live a righteous life, I gained the knowledge needed to create my own set of values and morals through my self-discovery journey.

Despite my middle school troubles, I tested high enough to get into a well-known high school where I made friends quickly. I also met a boy on the first day of school and became infatuated. Just as things seemed to be going well, our house was raided. I was in the basement exercising with my mother and sister when we heard a loud commotion, "GET THE ***k ON THE GROUND!" We did not think anything of it because my dad was the prankster in the family. After peeking around the staircase, I froze as a laser was pointed between my eyes. We were instructed to turn around, put our hands on our heads, and walk up the stairs backward. I was terrified that I would fall, and they would shoot me. We sat handcuffed at the table while they destroyed our house, ripping each and every poster off my bedroom walls as if there was a hidden safe behind the images of Chris Brown. This situation, combined with the prior harassment, led me to feel unsafe in my own home. So, I took solace in my relationship.

Over the next two years, the relationship blossomed. If you saw me, you saw him, and vice versa. I was so wrapped up in school and my relationship that I did not notice my household falling apart. Next thing I knew we were moving to Brown Deer leaving my dad behind. This was a big change as I had spent my entire life in that house. These sudden changes altered my mood, consequently affecting my relationship. My boyfriend and I broke up, so I decided to change schools. This was a fresh new start, being that no one at this school knew me. I decided to reinvent myself. I got this idea that I could be whoever I wanted as long as I believed it. This thinking method proved beneficial as my boyfriend and I rekindled our relationship, and I enjoyed my last year of high school.

By this time, I had dreams of becoming a chef, but my mother was adamant that I choose a career with more financial stability. She researched a couple of different professional fields and we decided on visual communications. Although I had been working since the age of 14, it was time to get a job that paid more than minimum wage, so that my boyfriend and I could move out. I started working for a captioning service where my job was to listen to personal phone calls and repeat what the speaker said. Six months into working at this new job, we relocated. We moved to a suburban area as the crime was increasing in the inner city. Our family and friends were not too happy with our decision to move far away, but it felt safe. Even though I was juggling school, the job, and being out on my own, I found balance. This good energy continued for about a year.

Our household was now struggling to make ends meet and this caused a lot of arguments. As a solution, I put my visual communications degree on hold and enrolled in cosmetology school. I chose this route because I was able to make money doing hair while gaining an education. The amount of change I was experiencing was taking its toll. The school workload, the hate speech endured at work, and the constant arguments at home were all too much. I began reading multiple books a week at work to provide a distraction from my everyday life. It got to the point where my reading followed me home as I just wanted to be anybody but myself. Cosmetology school took a turn for the worse when I started making extra money doing hair out of my house. I ended up taking my clients to my mom's house because it was an issue at home. Soon after I started doing an externship at a local salon, I realized that hair was not my future career. Subsequently, the smartest thing to do was to finish my visual communications degree.

The city I lived in had grown more and more violent by the year. It was not safe to go outside or even grab groceries from the local store. It got to the point where I only ventured out for work purposes because it was a necessity. I was still working at the captioning service when the first Black president was re-elected, which caused many disturbing conversations that affected my mental health. For months, my boyfriend would attempt to talk to me and ask questions only to be responded to by tears and empty eyes. I voiced my concerns to the supervising staff as well as the HR department and was told to hear it, repeat it, and forget it. This launched me into a deep sadness where I spent eight to 12 hours a day at my desk crying and contemplated ending my life. School was also added stress as it was my final year, and things were coming to a close. I ended up taking my troubles home with me, which influenced our decision to move back home with our parents. At this time, I decided to seek professional help and was put on anti-depressant medication.

Shortly after, my grandmother passed. She was the matriarch of our family and held everyone together like glue. We all seemed to unravel due to her passing. My mother took it the hardest; they were best friends. Being witness to my mom's pain without being able to help was hard to deal with. After that loss, my dear friend Ashtian Duane Barnes was gunned down in Houston on the beltway, by a Deputy Constable, for no reason other than his skin color. Not only did I lose a very dear friend, but I also watched him gunned down on a dashcam video which is still available online. The video shows my friend did nothing wrong, yet the officer was not charged for his murder. This hurt so bad that I had no desire to even be on this earth anymore. I stopped eating, drinking, and sleeping. I will forever be traumatized by this event. These losses changed me and ultimately affected my relationship.

One night, I browsed my cousin's Amazon account and saw a book in her cart that I was interested in—Emma Mildon's *The Soul Searcher's Handbook*. My mother, sister, and I chose to book a trip to Mexico as a farewell to my grandmother. I decided to bring the book along and spent quite some time in Mexico reading through it. The handbook introduced me to a whole new world of things I had yet to explore. I felt as if something was missing; I did not have a strong relationship with God and my family had never offered a sense of safety. *The Soul Searcher's Handbook* introduced me to the art of Tarot. On my first reading, I felt a deep connection as the cards knew things I had not told a soul. They advised me to leave my relationship and although it was hard, I booked a one-way ticket to Arizona and did not look back!

Jewlz's Old Way of Thinking – Negative Thoughts

Lack of Safety. Since I was a little girl, I always felt unsafe—unsafe in my home, unsafe at school, unsafe outside, and unsafe within my temple.

Pessimism. I never thought things would get better. There are these cycles that play out repeating themselves over and over again. I was stuck within this cycle, not able to see a way out. One of my favorite sayings used to be, "We gonna die anyways." I used it to justify my thoughts, feelings, the media, and life in general.

Jewlz's Old Reactions and Behaviors

Coping. To cope, I read books. I had read anywhere from five to ten books a week. I used reading as a way to escape my reality, if even just until the next call connects at work. It was my sense of freedom, my sense of hope!

Self-Harm. I have tried to commit suicide more times than I would like to admit, although I feel self-harm has more to do with putting yourself in a box restricted from growth than physically harming yourself.

Jewlz's New Way of Thinking – Positive Thoughts

Unlearn to Relearn. I began reading a number of self-help books in which I learned that there were deeper issues I needed to deal with. From that awareness, I had to accept where I was in my life and journey. I had learned so many things that were either working against me or simply did not serve me. It was time to start a process of unlearning in order to relearn.

Gratitude. A while back, I started practicing the principle of gratitude. When I wake up in the morning, before my feet touch the floor, I say, "Thank you, thank you, thank you!" When I have a negative experience, instead of immediately griping, I try to think of what I can learn from this experience. The Universe will send you test after test, and it is up to you to pay attention and work towards successfully completing them so that they would not keep repeating, thus stopping the unhealthy cycles in which we seem to constantly find ourselves.

Divinely Supported. Whatever it is that you need, whether physical, emotional, spiritual, etc., the universe will provide when the time is right. For me, that was a support system—the kind I sought in a family. The Divine Nine came at a time when I needed them most. I was reintroduced to my Father Ra, my Grandmother Ma'at, Mother Auset, and Spirit Guide Heru, to name a few. These divine beings have shown love and support, giving me the guidance I need to take on every day.

Jewlz's New Responses and Behaviors

New responses (behavior): Feelings and emotions that are generated by positive thoughts and how these new emotions encourage better behaviors.

Self-Care. I spent two entire years focused solely on taking care of myself. It was imperative to rebuild my relationship with my shadow that I had damaged throughout the years. I took her on trips, ran her baths, made her food, and rubbed her back, with the sole aim of being reunited again. I took care of her so well that she could not resist my Venusian charm. A wise woman once told me, "love begets love."

Self-Love. I started by showing myself love by reprogramming my thoughts. Each time I have a negative thought, I quickly replace it with three positive thoughts. When my feet are aching, I rub them. When I cook myself a meal, I say thank you. When I have a long day, I hug myself.

Self-Respect. I began a long journey of learning to say "no" and speaking up for myself. The quickest way to let yourself down is to fold on one of your boundaries. They are put in place for a reason, and being the peacemaker that I am, I have always shied away from holding on too tight to my boundaries. It was not until I took a trip to the East Beaches of Toronto and a man who resembled Leprechaun in the Hood talked about the value of *your truth* that I began even to consider freeing myself.

Jewlz's Restoration Tip

Restoration requires knowledge, sacrifice, and discipline. It is up to you and you alone to make healthy decisions as you will be held accountable for your choices. I have used my experiences and what I have learned on my 5-year journey to turn negatives into positives. I stand before you, the Master of my own UNIverse. I challenge you to become the master of your own UNIverse as well.

Jewlz's Definition of Success

To me, success is found in values, morals, and beliefs. Although I have multiple businesses and a budding career, none of that would be possible without the knowledge I have accumulated. That base of knowledge led me to develop my own system of righteousness.

Jewlz's Journey to Wellness Takeaway

I stand by the saying that knowledge is power; when you know better, you do better! The more I learned, no matter the topic, the more seeds were planted, and the more I grew. My takeaway from my journey to wellness is that it does not matter where you start or your destination, just that you have the courage to start. Secondly, putting time, effort, and intention into any area of your life is going to benefit you profoundly. I started a spiritual journey with the hopes of finding light in the darkness and ended up finding the light within me. It is safe to say I am no longer afraid of the dark; I welcome the discomfort, as there is no growth in comfort zones.

Jewlz Advises

My advice is for those who are afraid of the unknown, the darkness. You will never experience growth if you do not travel outside of your comfort zone. Some of my most rewarding experiences have come from stepping out in faith and trusting in myself. I recommend starting your journey of self-discovery immediately. No matter where you are in life, every version of yourself will require a new level of self-discovery. Blessings!

Journey to Wellness Practical Tool

Cognitive – Old Way of Thinking - Negative Thoughts
Instructions: Pause and take three deep breaths to clear the mind, then complete the exercise. List three negative self-thoughts you experienced during this chapter.

_____

_____

_____

_____

Emotional – Accepting Feelings and Emotions – Negative or Positive
Instructions: Pause and take three minutes to notice and connect with your feelings, then complete the exercise. Identify, list, and recite three emotions you are feeling at a particular moment. Be compassionate with yourself.

_____

_____

_____

_____

Cognitive, Emotional, and Behavioral – New Way of Thinking, Responses, and Behaviors
Instructions: Reflect on the questions throughout the chapter, explore new thoughts and desired changes. Rewrite the three negative thoughts listed above into positive thoughts.

_____

_____

_____

_____

Recite each rewritten positive thought three different times throughout the day. Remember to use a compassionate tone. Journal the times below.

_____

_____

_____

_____

Name three adjectives to describe how you felt after the positive self-talk exercise.

_____

_____

_____

_____

List three ways how you will think or respond differently to adverse challenges in the future.

_____

_____

_____

_____

PART SIX

Making Choices

Proclaim:

*Making conscious choices to change your thoughts
heightens self-awareness and provides the clarity
needed to change your outcomes.*

Visualize yourself swimming down the Mississippi River, the second-longest river in North America, 2,320 miles long. The flow is natural. The water collects small pieces of debris off the shores and rocks. The scattered pieces of waste accumulate until daunting heaps of waste surround you. To avoid directly confronting the discomfort of a new situation, you choose to go against the river's natural flow and start swimming upstream because you dread the confrontation that comes with growth and would rather return to infancy. Thus, you swim for days, weeks, months, and years on end, trying to recreate a blissful time in your life because you are uncomfortable in the new situation. Instead of adapting to the new environment, you seek to ease yourself of the discomfort by fleeing the scene.

In making choices and dealing with challenges, first, this soul-searching question is vital: How do you cope, confront, or ameliorate an unpleasant situation—by taking responsibility or passing the buck? Do you play the blame game when your coping skills are running empty? Suddenly the nearest individual becomes the targeted scapegoat. It was you who said "Yes" and dove into the river, but now it is no longer your fault; it is theirs. But may I deliver the candid truth: taking responsibility for your actions should not be an option, so sit in the mess that you created until you choose to change. Sit in the mess until you recognize the past is past (if it is a transient moment of pleasure behind you that you are yearning for), and no matter how hard you try to recreate that blissful moment, it is a lost opportunity, for there is no future in that past. You are bound to lie in this mess until you take the initiative to clean up what has accumulated since a mess cannot clean itself.

If I should continue being candid—and I must—then I have to admit that change is not always easy to achieve quickly. Even from the analogy that opened this chapter, it is evident that so often, people conceive the concept of change as if it is as simple as counting 1, 2, and 3. We commonly hear statements such as, "You need to change the way you think," "Just change how you respond," and "You should change what you say and how you say it." Alas, it is all easier said than done. It is important to note that change is not a light switch. You do not walk into a convoluted web and flick the button, and the "change" magically happens—going from darkness to light or vice versa. One purpose of my journey is to change maladaptive behaviors by using differential positive actions I deem appropriate and necessary. So do not beat yourself up if you feel like you cannot seem to bring change into your life yet. Not everyone can change themselves as easily as others—some need to go into deep reconstructions, just as I did.

Let us keep it real! Some of us get offended when change is suggested. Though adaptation is a common life skill, a lifestyle change requires breaking the primordial mold in order to build a better one. While it is easy to process change as though something is wrong. One has to think more positively and make a conscious effort to move forward with the possibility to change. And challenges should not deter you but prepare you. On average, it takes two to three months before a new behavior becomes routine, and depending on one's willingness and circumstances, developing new habits may take up to one year. In some situations, biological and genetic predispositions may warrant assistance with change by considering a combination of psychotherapy and medications to manage one's cognitive-behavioral outcomes. These options aim to stabilize chemical imbalances that may cause significant impairment to one's healthy functioning.

Again, I am well aware that change is not an easy task. However, to reiterate, I am confident that it is possible. When you have taken responsibility for your actions (and not playing the blame game), consider these other vital questions:

Have you identified a behavior you desire to change? What is it? Why do you desire to change it? (Desire begets change.) Do you feel professional assistance needs to be employed in your situation?

Some people cringe at the idea of asking for professional assistance. The stigma and perceptions associated with mental health issues, for instance, are barriers to explore and engage in treatment options. Results of various cultures that I have interviewed suggest that minorities are least likely proponents of soliciting aid in this area because it is viewed as a sign of weakness. And in this modern society of ours, too pent-up in its peril, not many people are willing to come across as weak. But like I stated in a previous chapter, we do not have all the answers, and individuals who are more adept at specific issues do surround us. If it is an area where we need help, please ask! Asking for help does not make us weaker than others. It actually strengthens us. If you become physically ill, you will seek medical attention, so why not seek mental health services when there is a cognitive imbalance?

In all honesty, for many years, I did not fully appreciate my abilities, worth, and value. Although I never digested the spell, "I'm not good enough," there were overwhelming moments of distress that caused me to feel that way.

During my first year at Georgia Perimeter College, I dealt with feelings and belief systems, believing I was neither smart nor intelligent. Nerve-wracking, I tell you. One of the required classes was United States History. I recall sitting in the third row from the left of the room and the fourth seat behind. My professor, a divorced chain smoker in his early 50s, was fervent about history. He talked about the Quakers, Founding Fathers, Civil War, Jim Crow, Industrial Revolution, Cold War, and so on. It was a lot of information, and at the time, I was not exceptionally thrilled about history. Math, health, and science were subjects of interest.

As weeks passed, the time came for our first quiz. Though I studied, I failed, leaving me devastated. A week later, he administered a 50-question examination, and again I failed. Throwing my hands up with disappointment, I could not comprehend receiving two failing grades consecutively. I studied, and I practiced. So, what happened? What went wrong? Those were the grueling questions I asked myself. After self-assessing and hitting roadblocks, I concluded that I had an undiagnosed learning disability. Consequently, I scheduled a consultation with my professor based on my process of elimination. During our meeting, I learned that the college did not have any resources to learn history better. For math, reading, writing, and science, the college provided tutors. But when it came to history–nada–I was on my own.

The professor offered a few suggestions based on his assessment, which I acknowledged, and on the next quiz, I received a C. At the end of the class, we reviewed the questions I answered incorrectly, and he offered additional suggestions. Again, as soon as I got home, I studied, reviewed, and practiced in preparation for the next examination. Bam! Another C. Guess what started happening? My grades improved, and my confidence and self-esteem increased. I thought and said to myself, "Self, if my grades are improving, it is a strong probability I do not have a learning disability." "Can I sustain the academic up-tick?" I wondered to myself. Thus, I continued meeting with the professor after each quiz and examination, and the change turned into the inevitable. I witnessed the "self" changing. Embracing the change fostered the changed man I am today.

D.B. Marshall's Definition of a Changed Person

A Changed Man or **Woman** *is the one who is astute and focused on a specific trajectory that makes the necessary modifications by introducing action-filled new approaches along the way in order to ensure and assure his/her happiness.*

By the end of the semester, I completed the course with a low B. It was a long, rough ride downstream in the Mississippi River against the current. But the zeal for change helped me earn a B. The untold truth, however, is: I am not a fan of B's. A's look absolutely stunning on transcripts, which also tends to boost my confidence. But when I saw the" B" next to *U.S. History*, it had the same emotional effect as an "A" would have, and I low-key screamed, "Hallelujah!" You see, when I received failing grades on the quiz and examination, negative thoughts immediately started mass-producing artificial information, transmitting false messages into my mind that I was a failure, that I was not smart, that I was not intelligent. But these ambiguities were far from the truth. The real issues consisted of two things. One, I had to change the way I studied. My review had to look different than it did with math, science, and health. Universal study approaches did not apply to subject-specific areas such as history. With history, understanding and connecting timelines, periods, names, and locations were crucial.

Two, I needed to take the initiative and ask for support. Sometimes resources are around us, but we must open our mouths in order to be fed. I urge you to develop a neighborhood, church, or community directory with a list of resources and make them readily accessible in unforeseen circumstances. It will enhance your life and the lives of others. Please understand that resources or resource channels come in many forms. They are not always monetary or tangible in nature. Some of the most valuable resources are intangible such as attentive listening ears, empathy, sympathy, and understanding. Intangible resources like the non-judgmental love of my family have guided and supported me through some tough times. As the saying goes, "People may not remember what you did or what you said, but they will always remember how you made them feel." Thanks to Maya Angelou for inventing this life-changing statement.

Talking about human resources of change and remembering Maya Angelou's words to that effect, I am compelled at this juncture to acknowledge a number of persons who have been tremendously instrumental to my transformation. A special thanks to Mrs. Van Beverhart, Mrs. J. Brogdon, Ms. L. Zephir, Mr. D. Safford, Mrs. Williams, Ms. D. Dykes (my Shonny), and Mr. M. Rouse. These are not only my superheroes, but they are also my authentic intervention soulmates. They evoked smiles and influenced away ugly cries. They complimented my strengths while dousing out weaknesses. When the thought of "not good enough" invaded my mind, they intervened with reverence and showed me that I was an exceptional person, a masterpiece. They made sure I understood that I could not be replicated or duplicated. These superheroes of mine hugged me in my imperfections so tightly until the imperfections changed to become the decoration, resembling the blessed stained-glass windows of Sainte-Chapelle in Paris, France.

That is right. My superheroes intervened with heroic thoughts. Collectively, they brought productive solutions to reverse unproductive thoughts. They saw amiable forces within me, even when I failed to acknowledge my expansive potential

144

capable of refining my growth. Although I could not see the infinite possibilities in myself, I realized the potential they saw was exactly what I saw in them: strength, tenacity, dedication, happiness, and vibrancy. Confused about why I saw these character traits in them and not in myself, I eventually understood precisely what they were seeing. While I was looking at them, it was actually me staring directly in front of a mirror, looking at my reflection the entire time.

Take time to self-assess and make conscious choices to change self-deprecating thoughts. Positive change can remove barriers and provide the clarity needed to close chapters and bridge gaps. When clarity happens, an awakening occurs. The growth represents the desire to do better, want better, love deeper, and become all you desire to be.

Awareness + Desire = Change

For change to occur, first identify the destructive habits in your personality that need shedding. Other times it may not necessarily be a habit; it can also be a person, an environment, or even a thing. Once the habit or influence is identified, start inducing change. To induce change is to visualize yourself in an environment or phase where change has been made. Imagine living a better and healthier life. Own the fantastic depiction that was just engraved in your mind. Picture and imagine every single detail of this new life. This will motivate the mind to create the actions to change. But it only happens when you are self-aware and when you desire to make the thought and content different from what it is or from what it would be if you did nothing. Once the oath is made and change is practiced, it will start to feel like a familiar friend. Embrace it with open arms. Keep at it until improvements are seen.

Now you have made the necessary modification to improve your life. Observe and journal how it improved for the better. Feel free to celebrate the wins. Even the slightest improvement calls for a celebration. And if you falter on the way,

LOVE'S PURSUIT: Journey to Wellness

do not beat yourself up. Let your family and trusted friends in on the changes in the atmosphere. You know, accountability is a vital factor in this process; it helps; if you start slacking, they can be there to redirect and support you along the way.

Be Aware. Show Desire. Change will Transpire.

Journey to Wellness Self-Discovery Reflection

What are the changes you desire to bring in your life?

_____

_____

_____

_____

What are the positive behaviors you desire to replace the negative ones?

_____

_____

_____

_____

Do you have the raw materials needed to bring about organic change? List them.

_____

_____

_____

_____

Who are the professionals who can help manifest your desire to change? Name them.

_____

_____

_____

_____

How will you make sure you are consistent on this journey of change?

_____

_____

_____

_____

Giving and Receiving

Smile
to yourself even when it hurts.
Dance
like no one is watching your stunts.
Give
to yourself the love you crave for.
Hope
like it is your entire life endeavor.
For the energy you broadcast will come back
When it has increased, and the same you attract.

Gratitude is another tool that will change your life. It can improve moods, increase hope and optimism, and improve intra- and interpersonal communication and physical health. So what is gratitude? Gratitude is the quality of feeling and being grateful and appreciative, not just for the big things but also for all things good. Many of us are excellent at giving gratitude by saying thank you. However, in my experience, I found it is quite difficult for many of us to receive it. I have met a plethora of individuals who cannot openly receive a compliment. They generally felt that a malicious agenda soon followed the heartfelt intentional gesture. This response can signify past hurt, abuse, fear, insecurities, and more. However, you possess the power to change the very things holding you captive. You will read about a heroic young man who had no problem extended gratitude to others in the upcoming story. One day, like all of us, life happened, and purpose forcefully knocked on his door. His smiles turned into frowns; the dancing halted because his record player was deemed technologically obsolete. He no longer had the physical strength to give, which left him emotional and emotionless. However, the act of receiving gratitude from family and others transformed his life. Readers, I introduce you to James Tolbert.

Physical Wellness

Meet James Tolbert

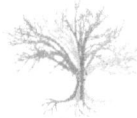

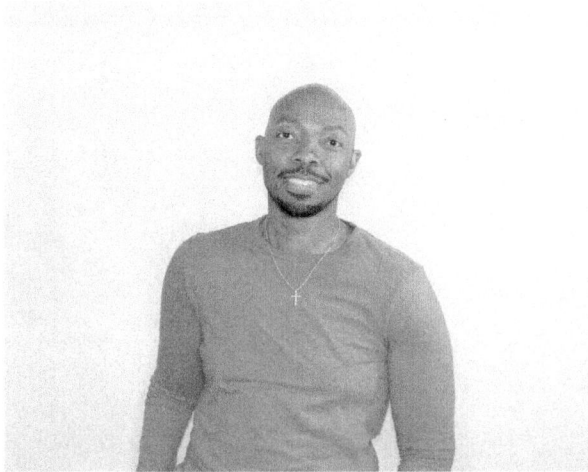

Proclaim:

"After I accomplished a goal, what's next?"

Introduction

Hi, my name is James. Born in South Georgia in the city of Rochelle in Wilcox County. "You can do it if you want to" was the basic mindset of all my family members. I mean, our psyche was conditioned from the cradle. Nevertheless, I was not a sociable person. That is neither to say that I hated people nor did I get myself at loggerheads with folks. The issue was that I did not fit in with the "normal" crowd because I was overweight (nearly 300 pounds), and therefore could not do much of what they did. With age, my condition led to self-consciousness and then insecurity. I camouflaged my insecurities by participating in simpler school programs like the Spanish club, Future Homemakers of America, and even Home Economics (the very thing I should flee; but oh no, I was always surrounded with food).

My childhood physical activities were limited. I did not have a wide variety of play or work. I believe it was because of the absence of a father or male figure to encourage me. Unfortunately, I was only nine years old when my daddy was murdered. Together, my mother and grandmother rose to the occasion of improvising fatherhood to meet my childhood needs. I accord them great kudos for a job well done. Yet, I began a journey in which I learned a lot: I finally started shedding pounds, and that meant I also started to gain the confidence to appreciate my real self. However, tragedy soon struck.

On January 7, 2001, I had an accident in my junior year in college at Fort Valley State University. While wrestling with a friend, I fell the wrong way and broke my neck, instantly transforming me into a quadriplegic at the age of 21. Paralyzed from the chest down and lost all functions of my hands, arms, legs, and other internal organs, I was terrified.

Despite being wheelchair-bound, I kept receiving spiritual and emotional pushes from my mother, grandmother, sisters, and other believers. When fall came, I decided to return to college. Confined in a wheelchair and taking a few classes, I attempted to inch my way back into society. I believe what helped spark the flames during that time was the words of my vocational rehabilitation counselor. He told me in clear terms that I could not make it in the field in which I was then majoring (that is, veterinary technology) because of my type of disability, that is, lack of body functioning, especially the hands. My counselor did not mean any harm, for he only followed the rules and evaluation. But being a person cut from my cloth, it seemed that was exactly the sort of naysay required to succeed. In May 2003, I proudly graduated with my degree a veterinary science and walked across the stage on my forearm crutches. After that long stride, I desired more. So later, I attended Armstrong Atlantic State University and worked as a substitute teacher. I proudly walked across the stage again on my crutches and graduated with a Master of Public Health in 2008.

The journey of regaining mobility with intense pushes in different directions—physically, mentally, and emotionally—has commanded my attention throughout the years. And at my present age, life is still a journey, a journey of rediscovery.

James's Identified Trauma, Challenges, and Barriers
Childhood Trauma, Denial, Rejection, Relationship Trauma, Not Good Enough, Body Image, Fear, Insecurities

James's Journey to Wellness Story
Oddly enough, my journey to wellness began after my accident. Although before I was actively losing weight and was actually succeeding, the success was superficial. I was losing weight for the world and not for me. But the first real trauma that plagued my mind before the accident was my father's death.

The loss of my father brought forth some guilt because it was a homicide case. It is weird, but I thought it was partially my fault. How foolish! I understood later that his death happened as a consequence of an altercation between two adults. Later, I learned that I was not responsible for the choices and behaviors of adults.

And then the accident happened. Complete physical immobility felt like a life-sentenced forever to an internal prison. Lying immobile in bed was not so bad until the medication—Baclofen—wore off, and my mind started responding to stimuli. Imagine your nose itching, and you cannot scratch it, or you want to change your position in bed, but you must wait until a nurse is

152

available to help you. I felt like a burden. When I regained my first movement (which was a toe), I made a resolution in my mind: *I got to have faith, have patience, pray, and keep going no matter the challenge or difficulty.* And my mother ensured I was reminded of that every day.

In 2001 it seemed as though my life reset by forces beyond the normal because next, I had to use a wheelchair. People who saw me probably saw only the exterior of my struggles, whereas, in reality, it was more interior. One may ask, "How is that?" Well, it is easy to rejoice when your body organs and tissues are functioning well and your expectations are materializing. But it is a different ball game to be grateful for the little "gains" such as, in my condition, tying my shoes, tilting my body without hurting myself, learning to stand, and other such small things. It takes conquering the ego (or shame, as the case may be) and past physical strengths and simply be grateful for each small degree of improvement made in the present. I had known how to push through obstacles, but many times those were for ignoble reasons, just so I could feel that I belonged among the "normal" people.

My wellness journey had to start on the inside, which made me want to go the extra mile, according to my own calling, and not just settle among the so-called normal crowd. I remember once sitting in front of a building, and on the left was a rehabilitation center and on the right was a fitness gym. Sitting in thought and praying, I mused that I could be content with rehab or get out of my comfort zone and join a gym where I knew it would be more physically challenging. Needless to say, I chose the gym, and there I was blessed with trainers who saw more in me than I ever did, and they pushed me beyond the mark of fear. Nowadays, confidence has increased, and I have developed a "try it" attitude. Now I attempt to do things in my physical capabilities again instead of what "*walkers*," as we call them, usually do.

James's Old Way of Thinking – Negative Thoughts

Doubt. Many times, I thought I could not achieve certain things I knew were possible. I have to admit, these thoughts still visit from time to time, but I have learned that the best way to get over it is to *try it.* For me, there are no more regrets if I can help it; instead, I try new activities, love new people, or travel more, even if it is alone.

James's Old Reactions and Behaviors

Feelings of loneliness often led to negative thoughts of "maybe I am not good enough," or "who would accept me for who I am," or "my disability is a hindrance to my future." All of these are reasons I became an expert at introversion. The emotional reaction reinforced my non-active behaviors and augmented "I am not good enough" thoughts at that 99999.

James's New Way of Thinking

My new way of thinking is a *"what's next?"* attitude, with prayer and spiritual guidance. Now I feel as though I can accomplish diverse milestones. And when I achieve them during that time, it is intoxicating—I want more. I desire more in life!

James's New Responses and Behaviors

Feelings of past accomplishments tell me that, "I did *that*, why can't I do *this*?" It is about trying something new, even when I feel" fearful," because it weirdly excites me. The emotional response encourages me to try a little harder. Before COVID-19, I was more active in the gym, wheelchair tennis, wheelchair rugby, and all. When corona blows over or is eradicated, I will return to these activities because they help create peace of mind.

James's Restoration Tip

Peace of mind and doing what *I want to do* is the thing! I never took time for myself due to the fear of disappointing others or being hurt. However, I realized that, hey, I will fall sometimes, but what matters is that I bounce back, mentally, emotionally, and physically.

James's Definition of Success
At this time in my life, I have accomplished so much. Success right-thriving day by day, looking forward to the next challenge, and knowing I CAN DO IT!

James's Journey to Wellness Takeaway
It is okay to fail as long as you try your best. Always remember there are options; as Claire Cook stated, "If plan A does not work, there are 25 more letters in the alphabet—204 if you live in Japan."

James Advises
Most definitely have a great support group of people, whether one or five, along with God's guidance. Remember to pause and reflect on how you have made it so far in life and feed those happy moments of peace. Take time for yourself. You cannot save the world or pour from an empty cup, so take care of yourself first. That way, you will have enough strength to help others along the way!

Journey to Wellness Practical Tool

Cognitive – Old Way of Thinking - Negative Thoughts
Instructions: Pause and take three deep breaths to clear the mind, then complete the exercise. List three negative self-thoughts you experienced during this chapter.

_____

_____

_____

_____

Emotional – Accepting Feelings and Emotions – Negative or Positive
Instructions: Pause and take three minutes to notice and connect with your feelings, then complete the exercise. Identify, list, and recite three emotions you are feeling at a particular moment. Be compassionate with yourself.

_____

_____

_____

_____

Cognitive, Emotional, and Behavioral – New Way of Thinking, Responses, and Behaviors
Instructions: Reflect on the questions throughout the chapter, explore new thoughts and desired changes. Rewrite the three negative thoughts listed above into positive thoughts.

_____

_____

_____

_____

Recite each rewritten positive thought three different times throughout the day. Remember to use a compassionate tone. Journal the times below.

_____

_____

_____

_____

Name three adjectives to describe how you felt after the positive self-talk exercise.

_____

_____

_____

_____

List three ways how you will think or respond differently to adverse challenges in the future.

_____

_____

_____

_____

PART SEVEN

Speak and Be

Proclaim:

Speak It!
Be It!
Be You!

One of the most difficult things I have learned in my 46 years of living is how to love me and be my authentic self. It is hard to figure, isn't it, how it took someone nearly half a century to know his soul and be comfortable in his mocha skin? Well, it encompassed coming to grip with the uniqueness of his or her own personhood. So what did I have to learn about myself? Well, the thing is, if I was not me, then who was I? I mean, if I despise who I am, who else then can I be? Am I to start pretending or mimicking and modeling someone other than me, disowning the imperfect perfect creation that I am?

From my story, I think self-rejection creeps in when one becomes more and more aware of one's peculiar flaws that are only known to themselves. It is weird and disturbing because you are familiar with your behaviors from cradle to old age more than anyone else. Then suddenly, this uncanny facet of your personality shows up struggling like shoulders-against-boulder up a steep hill. Wrestling with unfamiliar feelings of shame and guilt led me to believe something was inherently wrong. I found shame and guilt to be two good cousins. Shame, resulting from a negative evaluation of oneself, and guilt, rooted in regrettable deeds or words, often come together, intertwined. Things I may or may not have done or things I had failed at doing all caused moral infractions, which left me in a quandary. But all of this was soon about to change on my new journey of self-discovery.

On **Love's Pursuit:** *Journey to Wellness*, I am among the millions who struggle with these thoughts, behaviors, and emotions. I had to address the negative emotions that stemmed from primary and secondary trauma experienced in past personal and professional relationships. As I stated, these feelings were new as I did not encounter them up until my young adult years. I have crossed paths with some genuine people but also camped with talented manipulators. If you do not know who you are, then it is easy to become who or what they say you should be. But I urge you, my friend, allow no one to define you. Define yourself. What is the definition of you?

I am extremely, extremely grateful for my family and our values. Not once has my mother, father or grandmother suggested that I should be anything other than who I was, who I am, or what I am becoming. Within reason, my family permitted me to explore and discover what I had to offer in life. It was intentional and careless thoughts, managed and impulsive feelings, acceptable and unacceptable behaviors, good and bad influences, and more importantly, asking myself why. The only noun I was not allowed to question in our house was God. Even though the freedom to communicate and explore was the norm, it came with a cost, and sometimes that was a healthy price tag. But besides my family, my world was not one that was particularly morale-friendly.

I have always been curious about why it is so difficult to be exactly who we are naturally born to be? As I pondered on the "why," I observed that people and environments influence our personalities, identities, and behaviors. "I maintain that *nurture,* rather than *nature,* is the primary molder of personality," declared Nelson Mandela. So whether we admit it or not, we are products of influences. When we tend to talk of being influenced, we think of negative factors. However, for me, there are three dimensions of influence: positive, neutral, and negative. Influences can be negative (that is, dangerous), neutral (that is, impartial), or positive (that is, helpful). In the midst of inundating negative influences, our decisions should not be a question of if we should be who we are, but rather when do we choose to either operate in our birth name and birthright (that is, regain and maintain our originality) or separate ourselves from it.

Every year, I cruise with an amazing social group—SGL—and they have shown what laughter and love look and feel like. I joined their soul réjuvénation voyager as it was needed. Life was extremely rough, and I was immensely lost at the time. The group created a welcoming atmosphere that redirected my life forever. Love and laughter were rich in all the activities; it was almost tangible, even in the garments worn! I remain indebted to them and will always thank them for their generosity.

Every year, one of the group's activities onboard is speed dating. Now, I know what you are thinking, fix your mouth and do not say anything slick. Yes, I was single, searching, and patiently waiting to marry my person. Well, I really cannot honestly say "patiently waiting." And no, I was not thirsty either; my throat was just a little parched. Anyway, I met someone. Yes, I did. I introduced myself, "Hi, my name is Dammeon." Now when most people pronounce my name, they either say Damon, Damian, or Damien—never *Dammeon.* But here, when my name was repeated to me, I remember hearing Dammeon pronounced correctly for the first time. *Dam-me-on.* I was stunned. Shook. Even struck by lightning. Even my mother, father, and grandmother mispronounced it. There we were, hanging around, listening to the waves crash and reveling in the soothing midnight breeze on Deck 7. It was roughly 1:33 a.m. The sounds and vibrations rattled my soul like a triangle in E major in an Atlanta

Symphony at Chastain Amphitheater. It all magnified the magic of the moment, and I responded in utter awe. Furthermore, what was said next instantly created an unbreakable, everlasting bond that to this day cannot be undone—not by any mortal.

Do not let anyone speak or mispronounce your name. Every name, yours particularly, has purpose and power. Therefore, and since that day I am talking about, I kindly correct individuals who mispronounce my name. And each correction time is an opportunity to assert my identity, my self-asserted identity; for, to speak my name is to speak me. So I say, "Hi, my name is Dam-me-on, exactly how it's spelled." When I do this, they usually stop and look and say, "You're right." It is indeed pronounced exactly how it is spelled. As trivial as this may seem, it is quite significant. This was a milestone, for it was my first step in this journey to self-love and self-acceptance–Dammeon.

On November 4, 2018, at 10:40 PM, I was lying in bed, mulling over my to-do list one evening of the following month. This very instant, I received a random text from a church associate who I had recently met. The text message began by saying, "What does Dammeon mean?" I stopped and spoke to myself, "I know my name has power, but does it also have meaning?" Although I have heard people utter such statements throughout my life that everyone's name has a meaning and purpose, I never thought to search and discover the meaning of my own name. As you know, I have a relatively common name, but it is just that the spelling is vastly different. Do you remember those family road trips? When you finally crossed the state border into another rural town, stopped at the gas station, ran into the souvenirs section, hoping they had your name engraved on a keychain? I was always left disappointed every time. I found Damian, Damien, and Damon, but never Dammeon.

But back to the story at hand, the church associate texted the meaning. It read, "You're strong in material matters, determined, and stubborn." I paused and was like, *Hold up right here. Stubborn? Who's stubborn?* I knew they were not speaking of me. I read further, and it says, "You have a good business ability.

You are a good worker. You are steady and practical; a builder who takes responsibility well." I said to myself about these second descriptions; this *sounds more like it. Let us continue and see where this goes.* "These qualities may bring you to a position of authority and power." Authority and power... hmmm... sounds like there is leadership is in my blood. It further said, "You're a doer and down to earth. You're serious-minded, reliable, and have self-discipline. You also have a good power of concentration." I said to myself, *that sounds about right.* It also said, "You're bold, independent, inquisitive, and interested in research. You know what you want and why you want it." Well, that summed me up in a nutshell. Outside of my career, I did not always know what I desired but had a good comprehension of asking the question "why." The text also suggested that I understand the law of harmony and strike a balance between my life and those around me. Learning and understanding the meaning of my name acted as food for the soul. When I am me—Dammeon—there is an effortless sense of ease that kindly greets me every morning, afternoon, evening. With that, being me no longer felt challenging. Self-discovery was in a full transition toward transformation, which became effortless. The journey consisted of soul manifestations, visions, incremental gains, and revitalization—all because I deliberately chose to be who, what, and when, and had come to grips with the "why" and "how" of these choices of mine. This can be your manifestation, too. So, c'mon, join the journey to *Be it! Be You!*

Break here. Take a moment. Say this affirmation and repeat it two times:

Speak it! Be it! Be You!
Say it, again:
Speak it! Be it! Be You!
Again:
Speak it! Be it! Be You!

In relationships, I had often offered the most precious parts of me. Why? I believed that if I am in love, then I should be a representation of love. In my mind, love is abundant and is free—more abundant than water and freer than air; and love is healing itself. So why not love freely? Why do we have to earn love? Some treat love like a grocery item, stocked on shelves, with a price tag. What is your cost?

Here is another thought. My idea about love is based on my belief that I am a child of God who so loved the world that He gave His only begotten Son. That is a huge sacrificial offering of love, is it not? This is how I learned to love and desired to be loved. Well, this process does not work efficiently in the world we live in. Sometimes my vulnerability with others left one mess followed by another. Life became chaotic due to the premeditated malevolence of others. The strategic attack I experienced consisted of ego, greed, and deception. From this, I learned that not everyone would have my best interests at heart or capable of managing precious gifts, tender love, and care. Heck! Every time we choose to engage others, we take a risk and a leap of faith; and even then, it is wise to prepare ourselves for the unexpected because things are not always what they appear to be. As the saying goes, objects in the rear-view mirror may appear closer than they are. In life, mirages happen.

After running directly into brick walls and glass doors, I woke up, looked in the mirror, and realized that everybody does not operate like me. Talk about naivety. There are people who only saw a distorted image of me and did not see me for who I really was. In my mind, because I viewed agreements as legal bonds, it was difficult to terminate verbal, emotional, mental, and written relationship contracts. But alas, they did not share the same value system. It certainly suffered hurts because investments come with a price. I remember the one price that surpassed my threshold; the stock plummeted and left me emotionally destitute. When I said I do, I unknowingly agreed to potential chaos and turmoil when I signed the promotional for advancement. As a result, I chose to move into a small closet in an efficiency apartment, metaphorically speaking. That is right, a closet in an efficiency apartment. Imagine that if you can. I had gone from a world of exploration to a cubed box resulting in little to no imagination. Over time, the closet evolved into feelings of shame, embarrassment, guilt and felt more suffocating every day. After undergoing heartaches, disappointments, and blaming, I acquired knowledge that I had also played a role in the situation by choosing to say yes. I accepted and signed the verbal and written agreements. I did not investigate before investing. And having investigated, I would have said, "No, thank you." But I did not. I refuse to play the blame game; I instead take full responsibility for my part in the exchange.

When I understood this lesson, it was not long before my voice, value system, and confidence emerged from the ashes. Watch out now! I started to speak with an affirmed heart. I began wearing colors that spoke when I could not. For example, I wore pink, which fostered emotional healing, and green on days when I was not in a position to express compassion. After nurturing my heart, my eyes followed. Looking directly into them, I affirmed my soul daily with mantras and empowerment self-talks. Through this practice, I found love and an authentic fellowship, first with myself and then with others. I made allowances for my faults and forgave those who offended me, beginning with myself.

Once I extended an olive branch of compassion and grace, the true fellowship began to root, and I re-introduced myself to the "self"—my soul. I spoke into my life. I spoke into my existence. The chains of self-bondage were broken, and I moved out of the closet into the efficiency apartment. I have resumed the journey to wellness as the work has only just begun. When was the last time you gave serious and special attention to your journey of self-discovery? Self-exploration will allow you to discover hidden jewels, and they will modify your walk and talk. And, when times seem bleak, they will motivate and brighten your path.

Here is a word of caution: Do not explore for money, approval, social status, likes, or laughs. These reasons, besides being mundane, are a set-up for a beat down. Explore the world with the intention of strengthening self-fellowship and self-awareness. My process helped to understand some of my shortcomings, but more importantly, I began to understand my strengths. One of my greatest strengths is resilience. I have been through the worst of it and the best of it, but here I am, alive and still standing. That is what resilience is defined to be. I have lived half of my life, negotiated, and played around on the playground, even danced to the beat of someone else's drums, fearing relationship abandonment. No more! And, no, this does not mean selfishness or narcissism. It is simply a survival and thriving mechanism: withdrawal from toxins and tragedies. And the rewards for loving the "self" are unlimited.

I say to you: **Speak It. Be It. Be You.**

How can you expect individuals to understand you when you have not defined "you" for yourself? Begin right now, describe yourself with three words. This is you *speaking* it. Take a piece of paper out, write down features or qualities that you admire about yourself. Place them somewhere you could see them every day. Read them out aloud. Embrace these words. Demonstrate each word once a week. This is you *being it.*

Practice mantra meditations. This requires a clear mind. Sit with your back upright and close your eyes. Take three deep breaths. Hold them for three seconds or longer. Then let them out. With every breath that you let go, imagine all the negativity and toxicity your mind is harboring leaving the body. With every new breath inhale, reckon positivity and good vibes are entering the body. Now focus on your thoughts, but shut down any negative thoughts that may arise. It will take some time to stop intrusive thoughts, but you will master the technique with routine practices in no time. Think of progressive and positive things. Think of love. At this juncture, choose an affirmation from the

165

book and adopt it as a mantra. It will help overcome hurdles during your self-discovery, self-acceptance, and self-love life. Or you can also say any of these:

I am worthy of love.
There is someone out there specifically for me.

Truly believe in the words recited. Meditation fosters mindfulness, awareness, and calmness. It gives clarity of thoughts and opinions. It allows us to assess circumstances better and not fall victim to the same tactics of those who do not wish the best for you. It also empowers positivity; therefore, it will attract more positivity. Your aura will transform and light up whichever room you enter.

Journey to Wellness Self-Discovery Reflection

Are you comfortable in your skin? If yes or no, explain.

_____

_____

_____

_____

Thus far, what have you learned about yourself?

_____

_____

_____

_____

How can you own the imperfect perfect creation that you are?

_____

_____

_____

_____

Define you in three sentences or less.

_____

_____

_____

_____

List three family trips or experiences that allow you to be you.

_____

_____

_____

_____

What does your name mean?

_____

_____

_____

_____

Transformation

The rivers run into the sea,
And what becomes of the tributaries
Is accounted for in the ocean;
There the thoughts of the mind are called into question.
I urge you: reason and reconsider,
For you are what you ponder.

Why does your body atrophy in your youth?
Dust up your lazy butts and buckle up your boots;
For if your strength wastes away in young age,
What glory is there in your hair when it greys?

Your soul mummified today is reborn tomorrow.
Therefore knowing we will surely reap what we sow
And our harvests commensurate with the seeds planted,
We cannot but commit to purpose, taking nothing for granted.

We are perfectly imperfect. Say it with me. Ready. Set. Go. We are perfectly imperfect. Anyone who knows me knows I am also growing to reach self-actualization. Two to three years ago, suitors grew weary of my daily schedule. Until today, I work a full- and a part-time job, a full-time doctoral student, co-parent, and operate a business. Though I was upfront and transparent about my schedule and goals, someone once called me selfish. I was like, selfish? I looked at it from their perspective and saw how achieving my goals could be interpreted as selfishness. This is where I learned that when it comes to dating, I am consistently inconsistent. But, I am consistent. Now when I meet suitors, I make sure they understand I was made perfectly imperfect and strive to be consistent even though my life's purpose may cause inconsistencies. Caleb knows all about striving for perfection. He, like me, fought internal battles to answer questions to understand the "self" better. We consulted family, friends, communities, neighborhood, television, and faith-based institutions seeking answers and guidance to subside the anguish. Read Canaan "Caleb" Perry's ups and downs and the growth that followed.

Spiritual Wellness

Meet Canaan "Caleb" Perry

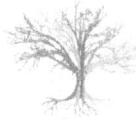

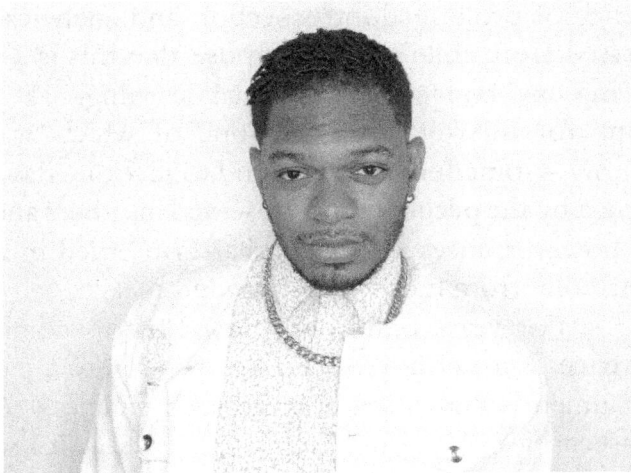

Proclaim:

Without every piece of a puzzle,
the picture can never be complete.
Guess what, you are a puzzle piece.

Introduction

Hi, my name is Caleb. Born in Champaign, Illinois, I was raised all around the world by a single parent. That "all around the world" of mine, however, was chiefly Cleveland,

Ohio. My mother, in raising my three siblings and me, imbued us with self-awareness; that way, we can be honest with ourselves as much as possible, and therefore extend the same grace to others. This fostered the culture of patience and support in the family, such that amidst disagreements (which you should always expect from kids), we could still demonstrate understanding and grace towards one another. This was the lifestyle ingrained in us from a young age. So, we knew from early nurturing that love transcends the superficial notion of feeling; we knew that love is principally a thing of the will (that is, decision) to act or react in a certain way for the good of people.

In hindsight, I could say with almost 100% certainty that this self-awareness upbringing supported my natural tendency of prolonged introspection and analytical mind that I possessed from childhood. I suppose that this is a subtle way of exposing my congenital antisocial learning. There were two reasons for this characteristic, one of which was underlying insecurity—something I was bound to face one day. I was usually intrigued by the peculiarities I observed in others and, at the same time, however, insecure about what I observed in me that made me different from most people around me.

For years I did not know how to communicate this difference. Furthermore, realizing that I was a gay male in an environment where there was no such example only deepened my insecurities. All along, I felt alone. Although I was not alone, in actuality, the feeling left me isolated. I learned that I was not alone. It was not until I realized in the ninth grade that others shared similar interests and ideas that I began the journey to self-discovery and self-acceptance. But first, I had to define myself respective to my faith. Questions like "What do I believe?" and "What does that mean regarding other areas of my life?"—and answering them—were pivotal.

The second is fear of rejection. In my youth, I developed many feelings that were primarily the result of uncertainties of myself. They included feelings of anxiety and hopelessness, which would later impact future relationships. I developed a fear of denial and rejection, always longing for a space to be fully loved one day—just as I am. Whether through an individual or an organization, I just wanted to feel like I belonged. But over the years, I have come to realize that true love is unconditional through many experiences and connections with many different people. And now, continually learning from the life of Jesus Christ, I aspire to love myself and others for real!

Caleb's Identified Trauma, Challenges, and Barriers
Denial, Rejection, Fear, Hopelessness, Insecurities, Not Good Enough, Relationship Trauma

Caleb's Journey to Wellness Story
Wellness is the state of optimal synergy. As previously mentioned, I found people and had relationships that afforded examples of love and belonging I thought I needed. This was the beginning of my journey to wellness.

To get to this point, I learned not to push through particular closed doors. I identified barriers that, instead of negotiating them, I simply took another path. I let certain ideas go. I let certain judgments go. And all these I consciously did. When I left home for college at 19 years old, for instance, I decided to let go of some previously taught thoughts about God and began developing a relationship for myself. I withdrew from man-controlled ideologies to explore self-awareness and self-understanding. It was sufficient that the Bible and most churches proclaimed the bottom-line of faith and reason for Jesus Christ: *unconditional love*. This became my philosophy of life, and I began applying it (the unconditional love) to develop myself further. I began to forgive and support myself in ways that promoted a sense of self. I opened up to God's grace and mercy, which granted me permission to witness how much God loves me, and consequently, how I could love others.

Caleb's Old Way of Thinking – Negative Thoughts

Some of the old thoughts that plagued my mind were: "I can't be good because of my sexuality," "I'm going to hell," "There is no hope for me, so why try to live, *right?*" "I don't know what I deserve if anything," and "How can I have been created without my choice and then made bad? —and why, if so?"

The only way I could react to these thoughts was to go and hide within. It contributed to keeping all thoughts and ideas in a protective, special place, rejecting them as unworthy to be recognized. And so I spent quality time with the one person who truly mattered—me. I did not think I could be valuable to others in any capacity. By these thoughts, I diminished the great work of God, that is, the development of self towards my purpose.

Caleb's Old Reactions and Behaviors

The emotions fueled the fear that "being as I am" would be detrimental for me and others. I had a tremendous amount of fear to live out loud, so to speak. So, I kept to myself. I went to work or school and came home to emptiness. I wrote—great ideas pumping in my head—but wrote ideas only to trash them sooner than later. I often gave up my dreams and aspirations, believing I could not and should not pursue them. Yes, I literally thought this way about myself.

When it comes to friendships...what were those? I did not have friends. Well, to be honest, I had friends but was not a friend. I did not see any value that others could have with me. Many people would communicate or interact with me, but that only made me nervous. I would not know what to say, or I would doubt what I wanted to say, and therefore say nothing. I constantly doubted my-self and questioned practical thoughts and good intentions.

Caleb's New Way of Thinking – Positive Thoughts

Now, in contrast to my past, I have fresh thoughts flooding my mind. Healthy thoughts are: "You are valuable," "You are worth being loved," "You are good and have great potential to be even better," "Jesus came for all, including me," "It is okay to be different," and "Someone can and will benefit from your experience and testimony."

Understanding the experiences of others who may (and should) look and feel different than mine and acknowledging the beauty of their lives and mine have allowed me to cherish and honor my own experiences, beliefs, and ideas. The security that comes with this reconciliation furnishes my mind regularly with new thoughts and innovations. And I continuously feel valuable. I now feel safe within my-self.

Caleb's New Responses and Behaviors
My life has turned around completely. I am almost an open book, so I share my experiences or ideas on topics that concern us as human beings. I can relate to other people's stories and accommodate, if not welcome, different perspectives. Communication and relationship are a powerful and significant part of life now.

Caleb's Restoration Tip
Being a great artist means nothing if no one frequents your art. Accepting all that I am has granted me the comfort to share my artistry. My heart and life are the art I share with the world. And I pray that this display of vulnerability allows others to find that same comfort of sharing with the world.

Caleb's Definition of Success
Success is the accomplishment of a goal or goals. The goal varies from person to person. However, achieving the set goal is a success.

Caleb's Journey to Wellness Takeaway
I have learned that we all want unconditional love. It is neither often given nor is it abundant in the world, but it is ultimately what we desire. We may try to find it in material things or think that it is present with people of affluence. Being imperfect, we

search for this unconditional love in other imperfect human beings. But in all these, we emerge disappointed. I have also learned that the unconditional love we are looking for resides within us, as deposited by God. Once we reach and tap into that love, it oozes out of our pores and impacts all those around us. The more this happens, the more normal it will be. Essentially, we reap from the trees or flowers of the seeds we plant in our environments.

Caleb Advises

I advise every person to focus on being true to self. Recognize and appreciate yourself in totality. Let go of weighing what only makes others happy to your own detriment. Find happiness, grant grace, and mercy, cut some slack, and grant yourself patience. When you genuinely do it for yourself, peace and spiritual wellness become yours.

Journey to Wellness Practical Tool

Cognitive – Old Way of Thinking - Negative Thoughts
Instructions: Pause and take three deep breaths to clear the mind, then complete the exercise. List three negative self-thoughts you experienced during this chapter.

_____

_____

_____

_____

Emotional – Accepting Feelings and Emotions – Negative or Positive
Instructions: Pause and take three minutes to notice and connect with your feelings, then complete the exercise. Identify, list, and recite three emotions you are feeling at a particular moment. Be compassionate with yourself.

_____

_____

_____

_____

Cognitive, Emotional, and Behavioral – New Way of Thinking, Responses, and Behaviors
Instructions: Reflect on the questions throughout the chapter, explore new thoughts and desired changes. Rewrite the three negative thoughts listed above into positive thoughts.

_____

_____

_____

_____

177

Recite each rewritten positive thought three different times throughout the day. Remember to use a compassionate tone. Journal the times below.

_____

_____

_____

_____

Name three adjectives to describe how you felt after the positive self-talk exercise.

_____

_____

_____

_____

List three ways how you will think or respond differently to adverse challenges in the future.

_____

_____

_____

_____

PART EIGHT

Elevate

Proclaim:

*I elevate my spirit and
bear my soul with confidence
amidst the chaos as this moment is pivotal.*

The past weeks were trying, and still so today. I am chartering new territory. As I write this book, my life is currently beset with overwhelming conflict and chaos. It is not out of place for doubts to fill one's mind in moments like this. I am talking about milestone changes and growth spurts, not minor challenges. The overthinking and overanalyzing now characterize my next action step. I feed distrust and expansion. Is this a sign to discontinue, pause, or continue with the process? However, in the midst of all these, I know deep down in my heart that this project is special, and the *Burgeoning Souls*, including the readers, deserve someone to invest in their personal growth, including their families' development. Such is the case for everyone resolute in this journey—there is always a spark of light (hope) to keep you afloat to sail against the torrents.

You must make peace with the uncertainties of life; at times, it feels exciting, but there are also times when it is uncomfortable. Surely, I am punting the boat on troubled waters. The sunset approaches, and night arriving brings perplexity, anxiety, worries, fears, and disillusionment. In these obscure times, it is hard to see someone or something for who or what it really is, making life more precarious for those lurking in the wilderness. That is how present and future struggles are when one is in the middle of a conflict.

But do not worry and do not fret; this journey is our rite of passage. Our faith will illuminate the dark paths, and the unknown will be revealed. The doubts are short-lived because this clarion call invigorates hope. Single-handedly, I invited passengers to travel together to higher ground. They are not aware that my original plans were rerouted to establish balance as they are now the yin to my yang. We are the two halves making a whole, the black, and the contrasting white colors, bleeding into one another due to the moisture-creating shades of gray. The grey represents neutrality, and our positive attitudes and willingness shift the opposing forces we denounced. Because we chose to take this journey together, our powers and gifts strengthen and nurture the hearts of millions.

The mission of **Love's Pursuit** is to invigorate Humanity with Humility, Hope, Happiness, and Honor toward wellness through the art of love, kindness, self-awareness, and creative expression. While still in this pursuit, our brands will epitomize the self-love on which I harp. Our future is destined, our future is bright, and our journey leads to awakening the true self, developing a robust economy, and filling emotional vessels with eternal love.

Pay attention and trust your intuitions. Stand for truth and live with integrity, which vindicates the character's nobility even without uttering a word. Take back the personal power given to others, for they have proven themselves unworthy. Go get your inheritance. It is time to choose the path that births gifts and ideas and observe unexpected, pleasant blooms in your life.

To you, my Wellness Enthusiasts:

There's no I in me,
because the me is we,
and without you,
there's no me to see the beauty,
I see in me.
We're one and great clan like doves flying over the sea,
I cannot survive unless you join me.
Accept my invitation, and let's monumentalize the occasion.
Because there's no celebration unless I immortalize your soon-to-be.
We journey in harmony, showing the world that love is you and me—WE.

– D.B. Marshall

"Let's Be the 'We 'that We are Meant to Be."

Journey to Wellness Practical Tool
Instructions: Journal how you can elevate yourself and others

PART NINE

Family Dedication Reflection

Dear **Love's Pursuit** *Family,*

Growing up, I did not understand why Ma was never home. It took the wisdom that comes with age to realize that she was the house's sole breadwinner. Furthermore, I noticed she worked two jobs, hence her usual absence. Although my stepfather was not as away from home as she, we depended on her for everything. And even though Ma was always working, she used to make ample time to be with her family and loved ones. When I was old enough to understand adult life, it was a wonder how she was always there for us regardless of her job constraints. To her, family was everything. Work was necessary, of course, but the family was a priority. It was for the sake of the family that she worked so hard in the first place. I remember Ma always planning something for the entire family: from beach days to birthday parties, Halloween parties, and so forth.

    No, Ma was not a passive mother. She knew her purpose of true motherhood to everyone in the family: to care and to discipline. For example, she did not allow us to do much outside the house, like go to parties or sleepovers. To compensate for that, therefore, she used to bring parties or sleepovers to our home. Now that used to drive me crazy, thinking I could never go anywhere. She never explained why, and when she said no, it was just "no"! But in retrospect, I sit back and express gratitude for her not giving us that leeway. Only now are my eyes opened to the happenings of those days—where children went missing or were sexually abused. Ma's love and sagacity, shrouded in a façade of sternness, saved us. Today, I really appreciate that.

     If our childhood were a garment, it was not particularly smooth. We had rough patches. It was not easy. But it was not bad enough to break our family's spirit, as it could have. We weathered the storms. Every obstacle we encountered made all of us more robust, especially Ma. And this is all because of her. Yes, she made sure we got the basic needs, such as food in our stomachs and clothes on our backs; besides the mundane, she inculcated many morals and great values. For instance, she made us understand that though we did not have much, we did have each other. She would always say to us, quite firmly, "You (the siblings) have to stick together because you are all you got." That has remained in my mind like nuts and bolts. I used to think to myself that we have other family members—cousins, aunts, uncles, and grandparents—but now I truly understand what she meant. I see families that feud with their brothers and sisters and go weeks, months, and even years without talking to one another. Not us; we are very close because of the instilled family values. When one got in trouble, we all got in trouble in solidarity. Ma taught us so. And to date, even while we are living apart, she is always there whenever I call. I thank God for her.

     Looking back over my childhood, I would not have it any other way. I was drilled on so many issues. I learned that you have to struggle for your family no matter what. But apart from providing for the family, I must instill morals and values in my own children and never tolerate certain behaviors from them. As I get older, I pray that I live out the legacy of my mother more and more and become a great mother and grandmother, just like her.

– Chantell

*Dear **Love's Pursuit** Family,*

Growing up I was always told to be there for my siblings because family is everything and to cherish every moment. I never really understood the meaning in depth back then. So, when I was asked or told to do chores, I did. Like the time I was told to clean the kitchen and fell asleep without doing so. My mother came home from work around eleven o'clock at night and saw that I had not cleaned the kitchen and woke up the entire house, furious. That was the only time that happened. I felt terrible about my mom waking my brothers and sister that night because of my laziness. After seeing how my siblings suffered for my irresponsibility, I told myself, "This can never happen again!" But not all my cherished moments reflected laziness.

So, my siblings and I loved musicals growing up. Our favorite musical movie was Little Shop of Horrors with Tisha Campbell, Tichina Arnold, and Michelle Weeks. We all decided to give my mother and grandmother a show on Mother's Day. We invited all the family members to the performance as well, which I can say was so much fun and memorable. At the end of our performance, everyone stood up and applauded loudly. As we smiled and waved, giving thanks, I noticed my mother and grandmother crying, filled with happiness. Seeing them overjoyed from our performance also caused the tears to roll down my face. But that is not the last time I cried from a beautiful, memorable moment. Now, this cherished moment was a real tearjerker.

The birth of my son is the most cherished moment in my life. I knew for a fact this moment in my life is the number one top pick of all time. When I can repeat the date, time, length, and weight just like it was yesterday. It was October 5, 2011, at ten o'clock at night, when my contractions started. I barely held my composure once the contraction pain kicked in. My mom came over to support me in this time of need.

I kept telling her, "Let's go to the hospital because it is time." She replied with, "nope, not time yet." I waddled away headed back to my room, moaning loudly in pain. That continued for over three hours, and it felt like an eternity. Then finally, I heard mom yell out, "Okay, it's time

185

now!" I rolled out of bed and put my slippers on, and headed straight to the door. I did not realize I was leaving her until I heard, "Hold on, do not leave out by yourself."

Once we arrived at the hospital, the staff were waiting outside with a wheelchair. They took me upstairs to registration and the assigned room. The nurses prepped me for the spinal tap, and at 5:30 in the morning,g I experienced my most cherished moment. My son was born. As I held my creation, I realized cherishing life through moments is what life is all about from my point of view.

– Tavon

Conclusion

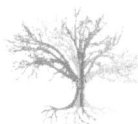

Proclaim:

The Mind – What I AM Thinking,
The Body – What I AM Doing,
The Soul – What I AM Developing

Having gone through these moving, intimate stories and their profound lessons, we hope that each wellness section motivated and inspired you to connect with the "self" so that tomorrow brings a state of hope. I have incorporated the tools and resources to jumpstart the necessary steps to a lasting, fulfilling life. Throughout the book, we have asked ourselves some difficult questions and challenged unproductive thought processes; however, it is only just the beginning. Set aside two to three months to adhere to and apply the recommended actionable steps. This allotted time is solely for your soul development, which is an investment in your healing and wholeness. As the soul develops, awareness, laughter, smiles, self-love, and empowerment also increase and develop. It is crucial to pay attention with the intent to nurture your mind, body, and soul.

The Mind *is what we are thinking.* Take heed to all thoughts (cognitive), both negative and positive, and streamline them. Life steers in the direction of your dominant thought, "for as he thinketh in his heart, so is he," Proverbs 23:7 reads. Mind the information that crosses your path. Filter them. Discard those that are judgmental, discriminatory, and harmful. Receive, absorb, and digest those that affirm, validate, and confirm, as it is a conscious step to eradicating negativity. Understanding that which does not make for peace, progress, and fulfillment is negative and must be deleted from your mind. The good you visualize when you close your eyes is the good that lies deep within you. Greatness begins with the simple thought of seeing yourself bigger than what you are today. What are you thinking right now?

The Body *is what we are doing.* The world we live in is the world of mortality; therefore, we use our mouths to speak (the behavior/action) affirmations to manifest our desires. Our bodies are action temples. It is in consistent movement that we achieve high performance. Henceforth, an excellent reason why it is important to keep a hale and healthy body. The Greek philosopher Thales put it this way:

"What man is happy?
He who has a healthy body,
A resourceful mind and a docile nature."

The Soul *is what we are developing.* The mind and body are in constant movement and developing the soul's (emotional energy) journey. What you choose to learn and apply will determine your life's path. Each question asked and answered

188

builds a comprehensive blueprint guided by the spirit in its wholeness. Self-awareness will delete erroneous thoughts making room to affirm exactly who you are and who you are destined to be. Soul development encourages you to enjoy the creative being you were born to be. If someone dares you to live in their box, it is likely that their box is located in the petite or young adult sections. And your dream is too big to fit in those areas. Ask them to point you to the big and tall or plus size section and find what looks good on you. Your purpose, dreams, or destiny will not catch everyone's eyes; but, you only need the right pair of eyes.

Here is a basic tenet to follow. External situations, interactions with other people, and negative events are not responsible for your bad moods, problems, and behaviors. When we can accurately calm situations without distorting reality, judgments, or additional fears, we are better able to know how to respond appropriately to feel happier in the long term. It is our own reactions to events, our "interpretations" of events that are under our control that end up affecting the quality of our lives.

Now it is your time to love and live happily! Let us establish new standards and re-establish a new personal order inclusive of revised tasks, values, beliefs, and morals. **You are worth it!** We are so delighted that you chose us to take this journey with, and we look forward to seeing and hearing how the book inspired your *Journey to Wellness*. Please share your stories on our social media platforms *@lovespursuitatl*, as you may be featured in our next wellness project in a city near you. Your journey starts here, starts now.

Oh, and by the way, if no one has told you that they love you today, please allow me to be the first: *I love you!*

Directory

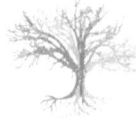

All in One Tax Services, LLC
www.Alln1taxjw.com
Facebook: All in One Tax Services/Credit Repair

Caleb Perry World
www.calebperryworld.com
Facebook: calebperryofficial
Instagram: calebperryworld
Twitter: calebperryworld

Good Karma Coffee House
31 N Avondale Rd
Avondale Estates, GA 30002
goodkarmacoffeehouse.com

Love's Pursuit, LLC
www.lovespursuitatl.net
Facebook: lovespursuitatl
Instagram: lovespursuitatl
Twitter: lovespursuitatl

Platinum Concierge-JW
www.Platinumconciergejw.com

Facebook: platinum concierge-JW
Instagram: platinum_conciergejw

SGL CRUISE
www.sglcruisecruise.com

SKNBRAND
www.SKNBRAND.COM
Instagram: SKN.brand
Facebook: Rashad Terry

SunGoddessBruja
www.sungoddessbruja.com
www.themoodypool.com
Facebook: sungoddessbruja
Instagram: sungoddessbruja

Urban Grin
962 Marietta St, NW
Atlanta, GA 30318
urbangrindatlanta.com

WERU Radio
www.weruradio.com

YNOTT Foundation
www.YNOTT.org
Instagram: mrynott
Facebook: edwardmrynottdrake
Twitter: mrynott

Zetta Nicole Girls Corporation
www.Zettanicolegirls.org
Facebook: zetta Nicole 'Girls
Instagram: zettanicole_girls

About the Author

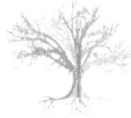

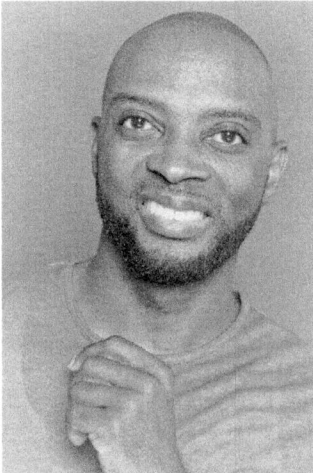

On October 1st, 2018, D.B. birthed **Love's Pursuit** out of emotional hardship, love, forgiveness, and spiritual enlightenment. In a robust effort to impact lives across the world, he has dedicated his heart, experiences, time, gift, talents, and more importantly his voice to uplift others through community advocacy and support. In addition, he became an Independent HerbaLife distributor to help others achieve their physical wellness goals. D.B. is truly a champion for invigorating humanity, hope, and happiness of those around him.

Even before entering his doctoral program in Social Work, D.B. devoted himself wholeheartedly towards the betterment of others in terms of self-confidence, attitude towards life, and overall wellness. His work with numerous charitable organizations including the American Association of Kidney

Patients (AAKP) Ambassador, Big Brothers Big Sisters program, and AAKP Patient-Centered Outcomes Research Institute Dissemination Award on peer-to-peer mentorship—as well as other community-focused pursuits—saw him develop a kinship with people from all backgrounds. His passion continues to grow, fueling his motivational and inspirational speaking pursuits, advocating for noble causes while capturing the hearts of thousands in the urban community on his wellness radio show titled "Wellness Wednesday" on WERUradio.com and podcast titled "The S.A.N.E. Project" on most podcast platforms. Today, that passion is stronger than ever; his honest devotion to humanity sits at the core of **Love's Pursuit** and continues to positively change and impact lives globally.

Education and Certifications
Doctor of Social Work (ABD), *Capella University*

Master of Social Work and Leadership Certificate, *Western Kentucky University*

Bachelor of Social Work, *Georgia State University*

Associate of Arts Early Childhood Education, *Georgia Perimeter College*

Wellness Coaching Services

SCHEDULE A CONSULTATION

The initial consultation is a scheduled 30 minutes with a wellness coach to discuss lifestyle concerns or obstacles. A brief Q & A will help determine if your needs are suitable for the wellness coach and company.

INDIVIDUAL WELLNESS COACHING

Individual wellness coaching sessions are 60 minutes. These sessions create a space to reconnect, remember, and reflect on your personal journey. It also is a space to receive feedback to determine the next action steps to reboot and achieve desired goals. The coaching sessions will: Help identify and decrease negative thoughts | Help increase positive thoughts and emotions | Help identify and develop strengths and talents | Help develop a sense of hope and inner light | Provide encouragement to live as well as be thoughtful and positive | Enhance goal setting, goal striving, and goal thriving skills.

GROUP WELLNESS COACHING

Group wellness sessions are 120 minutes. The group sessions are a safe, open forum guided by themes or topics that seek awareness, understanding, and support. Wellness groups consist of three or more participants with a wellness coach to discuss life and lifestyle concerns or obstacles. The group coaching sessions will: Help to normalize the theme or topic |

Help to develop a sense of hope | Help understand and cultivate a sense of happiness and wellness | Help to provide appreciation and celebrate incremental gains, activities, and accomplishments | Provide encouragement to maintain positivity and optimism.

References

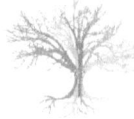

Ahmed, R., Bruce, S., & Jurcik, T. (2018). Towards a socioecological framework to support mental health caregivers: Implications for social work practice and education. *Social Work in Mental Health*, *16*(1), 105-122.

Brown, J. D. (2010). High self-esteem buffers negative feedback: Once more with feeling. *Cognition and Emotion*, *24*(8), 1389-1404.

Barok, S. (2016). Did you know…you have between 50,000 and 70,000 thoughts per day…Retrieved from https://www.huffingtonpost.co.uk/shahilla-barok/did-you-knowyou-have-betw_b_11819532.html?guccounter=1&guce_referrer=aHR0cHM6Ly93d3cuZ29vZ2xlLmNvbS8&guce_referrer_sig=AQAAAAyq2FYbIAhiuY7uCXrjYkClcPjkAMMWTm6b8Qe2gCS81Ss-9ptguu5kvxswAC6IkxZqKojpwCMgm4uQLOZszWmIhNuZYSM9lPLwTjNJKPiWlKW4bkxCNtoTjoqhEmEiyoJKfn02a9igWWK1RstKCZsXqsA5Y22R85-8W9VQ5GTS

Bussolon, S. (2017). *What is cognitive-behavioral psychotherapy?* Retrieved from http://www.neuropsy.it/psicoterapia/cognitivo_comportament ale/03.html

Chakhssi, F., Kraiss, J. T., Sommers-Spijkerman, M., & Bohlmeijer, E. T. (2018). The effect of positive psychology interventions on well-being and distress in clinical samples with psychiatric or somatic disorders: A systematic review and meta-analysis. *BMC Psychiatry, 18*(1), 211.

Chapman, G. D. (1992). *The five love languages.* Chicago: Northfield Pub.

Exploring Your Mind. (2020). How to turn negative thoughts into positive ones. Retrieved from https://exploringyourmind.com/turn-negative-thoughts-positive-ones/#

Federal Trade Commission. (n.d.). *Consumer information.* Retrieved from https://www.consumer.ftc.gov/

Food and Drug Administration (n.d.). *The new nutrition facts label.* Retrieved from https://www.fda.gov/food/nutrition-education-resources-materials/new-nutrition-facts-label

Greenberger, D. (2015). The link between cognitive behavior therapy and positive psychology. Retrieved from https://beckinstitute.org/the-link-between-cognitive-behavior-therapy-and-positive-psychology/

Keenan, E. K., Limone, C., & Sandoval, S. L. (2016). A "just sense of well-being": Social work's unifying purpose in action. *Social Work*, 1-10.

King James Bible. (2017). *King James Bible Online.* Retrieved from https://www.kingjamesbibleonline.org/

Muroff, J., & Robinson, W. (2020). Tools of Engagement: Practical Considerations for Utilizing Technology-Based Tools in CBT Practice. *Cognitive and Behavioral Practice.*

Pänkäläinen, M., Kerola, T., Kampman, O., Kauppi, M., & Hintikka, J. (2016).

Pessimism and risk of death from coronary heart disease among middle-aged and older Finns: an eleven-year follow-up study. *BMC Public Health, 16*(1), 1124.

Stefani, A. (2020). *Types of psychotherapy.* Retrieved from https://www.adrianostefani.it/articolo-psicologia.php?id_art=52&nws=3

Tovian, S. M., & Palomares, R. S. (2020). Clinical Applications of Cognitive Behavioral Theory of Personality. The Wiley Encyclopedia of Personality and Individual Differences: Clinical, Applied, and Cross ‑ Cultural Research, 37-53.

Yapan, S., Türkçapar, M. H., & Boysan, M. (2020). Rumination, automatic thoughts, dysfunctional attitudes, and thought suppression as transdiagnostic factors in depression and anxiety. *Current Psychology*, 1-17.